Dedication

To Jesus Christ. My Lord and Redeemer.
Finally... I am dedicated to You as You are to me.
Thank you for unlimited forgiveness and undeserved favor.

Acknowledgements

Rosanne, my wife.

You have stood by me and with me. If ever anyone wanted to meet the guy that has a wife who is truly his anchor... his "true north"... the guy that "smiles on the inside" because of her... I'm that guy.

My Children.

My persistent hope is that all of you will come to know Godly abundance as I have seen it come into my life. I also hope, as I continue to grow as a father, that you will be proud of me, as I relish the thought of you.

Donna Ferri and Paul Mueller.

Thank you for giving me the opportunity to work with you.
When I came to you, it was my last attempt to stay involved in the musculoskeletal arena. I had all but given up. You changed my life.

TABLE of CONTENTS

INTRODUCTION

Diagnostic ultrasonography as a general medical imaging modality has made very great advances in the last 10 to 20 years within the medical profession. Now, appearing on the horizon, is the more frequent application of diagnostic ultrasound to image musculoskeletal structures and the extremities of the body.

"Ultrasound imaging is not a passive push-button activity; rather it is an interactive process involving a sonographer, patient, transducer, instrument, and sonologist. Understanding the physical principles involved contributes to the quality of medical care involving diagnostic sonography."

This manual is intended to provide an introduction to musculoskeletal scanning protocols of the extremities, and hands-on use of diagnostic ultrasound.

The protocols presented are intended to provide a foundation from which physicians and technologists can develop more advanced ultrasound scanning abilities through education and experience in musculoskeletal ultrasound.

Sonography's unique real-time capability which permits examination during movement, and allows guidance of biopsy needles, combined with the exquisite resolution of state-of-the-art scanners and high-frequency transducers, makes musculoskeletal sonography a powerful tool for diagnosing abnormalities of the soft tissues. Musculoskeletal sonography has been underused in the United States because of the availability of magnetic resonance imaging. However; sonography can provide diagnostic information for only a fraction of the cost. In this era of cost containment in health care, musculoskeletal sonography should be the first examination technique for many pathologic conditions of the soft tissues.

I feel confident that these protocols will provide physicians information to improve evaluation and treatment of patients through the valuable diagnostic information obtained from the images.

Suggested Guidelines
Basic Musculoskeletal Anatomy
Normal Mean Values

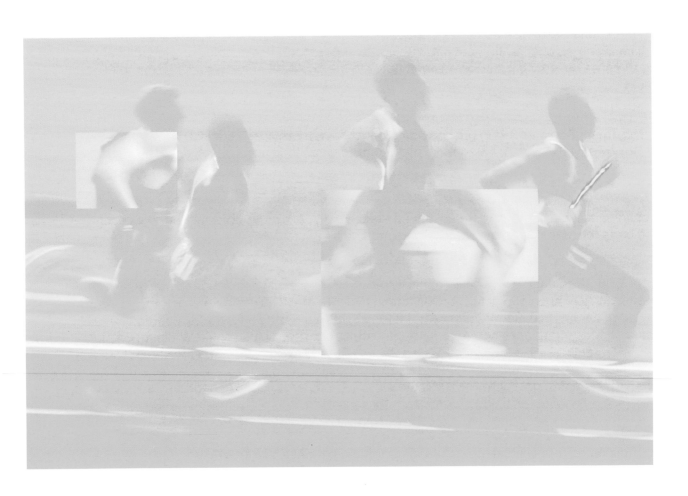

SUGGESTED GUIDELINES
FOR MUSCULOSKLETAL SONOGRAPHY

Equipment Selection

Musculoskeletal structures are long, striated and many times layered tissues. Due to the striated morphology of these tissues and their superficial location, high frequency, linear array probes are best suited for this application. It is recommended that no less the 7.5 MHz probes be used for musculoskeletal examinations of the extremities. Ideally, 8.0 MHz *and above* provide the highest resolution.

As in all ultrasound examinations, *proper technical settings are vital* to the diagnostic value of the images. Musculoskeletal images require adequate grayscale. Limited grayscale can lead to diagnostic challenges. Refer to the manufacturer of your equipment and their specific guidelines for optimal image settings.

Probe Placement

It is very important to maintain accurate probe placement in musculoskeletal sonography. Due to the close proximity of several distinct structures in a small area, a slight displacement of the probe can produce inaccurate images. If the image states it is a "midline" image be sure to be as close to midline as possible.

Image Orientation

Image orientation is consistent throughout the manual.
Regardless of right or left.
***Longitudinal views*: left side of the image is cephalad.**
***Transverse views:* left side of the image is the PATIENT'S RIGHT**

Tips For Technicians

Set your machine for proper grayscale.
Almost all images have the bony landmarks to be identified. Visualize the bony landmarks, and the surrounding soft tissue should be visible.
Labeling of images in this manual are *merely suggestions*. Feel free to establish labeling of images that are best for your facility. Take care to not make abbreviations too short to cause confusion.

Suggested Exam Protocol

The photographs in the manual clearly indicate patient and probe positioning. All examinations do not need to be bilateral studies that include identical images.
It is not necessary to perform all images described for each extremity in this manual on every examination. Images may be performed specifically in the area of complaint.
However, we recommend no less than 6 images per exam. 3 transverse images and 3 longitudinal images.

BASIC NORMAL MUSCULOSKELETAL ULTRASOUND ANATOMY

The following is a very basic introduction of normal musculoskeletal anatomy on ultrasound. In-depth knowledge of normal and abnormal musculoskeletal anatomy on ultrasound examination is available in textbooks that are currently available. This is provided as the most basic and fundamental introduction to allow scanning to progress more quickly.

SKELETAL MUSCLE

On longitudinal views, the muscle septae appear as bright/echogenic structures, and are seen as thin bright linear bands. On transverse views, the muscle bundles appear as speckled echoes with short, curvilinear bright lines dispersed throughout the darker/hypoechoic background.

FASCIA

Fascia is a collagenous structure that usually surrounds the musculotendinous areas of the extremities. The fascia is then encompassed by subcutaneous tissue. Many times, the fascia is seen inserting onto bone, and blending with the periosteum. Normal fascia appears as a fibrous, bright/hyperechoic structure.

SUBCUTANEOUS TISSUE

Subcutaneous tissue is isoechoic(equal brightness) with skeletal muscle. The difference between subcutaneous tissue and skeletal muscle visualized on ultrasound is the septa do not lay in lines or layers. More conspicuously; a thick, continuous, hyperechoic band usually separates subcutaneous fat from muscle.

CORTICAL BONE

On ultrasound examination, normal cortical bone appears as a continuous echogenic line with posterior acoustic shadowing i.e. it is black.

PERIOSTEUM

Occasionally; a thin echogenic line running parallel with the cortical bone is demonstrated on ultrasound. This is likely the periosteum however; in normal situations, periosteum is not visualized by ultrasound. Injuries to the bone, especially those damaging the cortex, periosseous soft tissues, and periosteum will produce a periosteal reaction, which is visible.

TENDONS

A normal tendon on ultrasound examination is a bright/echogenic linear band that can vary in thickness according to its location. The internal echoes are described characteristically as having a fibrillar echotexture on longitudinal views. On ultrasound the parallel series of collagen fibers are hyperechoic, separated by darker/hypoechoic surrounding connective tissue. The fibers will be continuous/intact. Interruptions in tendon fibers are visualized as anechoic/black areas within the tendon. Tendons are known to be anisotropic structures.

Anisotropy: An / iso / tropy. To not have equal properties/characteristics/ appearances on all axes. The property of being directionally dependent. Produced when the probe is not perpendicular with the structure being evaluated.

Most common artifact in musculoskeletal ultrasound.

LIGAMENTS

On ultrasound examination, a normal ligament is also a bright echogenic linear structure. However; ligaments have a more compact fibrillar echotexture. Individual strands/fibers of the ligaments are more closely aligned. Ligaments are composed of dense connective tissue, like tendons, but there is much variability in the amounts of collagen, elastin and fibrocartilage within a ligament, which makes its ultrasound appearance more variable than tendons.

PERIPHERAL NERVES

High-frequency transducers allow the visualization of peripheral nerves that pass close to the skin surface. Peripheral nerves appear as parallel hyperechoic lines with hypoechoic separations between them. On longitudinal views, their appearance is similar to tendons, but less bright/echogenic. On transverse views, peripheral nerves individual fibers, and fibrous matrix present with multiple, punctate echogenicities (bright dots) within an ovoid, well defined nerve sheath.

BURSAE

In a normal joint, the bursa is a thin black/anechoic line no more than 2 mm thick. The bursa fills with fluid due to irritation or infection. Depending on the extent of effusion, the bursa will distend and enlarge, internal brightness echoes are inflammatory debris.

NORMAL MEAN VALUES
UPPER EXTREMITY

*Biceps Tendon Cross- section = 3.0 – 3.5 mm ↕

*Supraspinatus Tendon Thickness = 4.6 - 6 mm ↕

*Subscapularis Tendon (transverse probe) = 4.2 mm ↕

*Critical Zone= 1cm proximal from SSP attachment

*Sub- Deltoid Bursa = 2mm or less ↕

*Rotator Cuff Interval (SSP and/or SCP) = 3mm ↔

*Humeral Head Cartilage Below SSP = 0.8 mm ↕

*Humerus—Acromion Distance = 10.9 mm ↘

*Anterior Glenoid Labrum = 3mm

*Ulnar nerve Cross -section = 7.5mm ↔

*Median Nerve Cross- section (proximal to carpal tunnel) = 9mm ↔

*Extensor Carpi Ulnaris Tendon (transverse probe distal to ulna) = 5.4 mm ↔

*Index Finger Flexor Tendon (transverse probe, volar)= 6.4 mm ↔

*Quadriceps Tendon thickness = 4.9 – 5.1 mm

*Suprapatellar Bursal _thickness_ (longitudinal probe) = 2.5 mm ↕

*Suprapatellar Bursal _length_ (longitudinal probe) = 19.5 – 22.5 mm

*Deep Infrapatellar Bursa sagittal thickness (longitudinal probe) = 2.7 mm ▶

*Patellar Tendon transverse thickness (transverse probe) = 3.0 – 3.4mm

*Patellar Tendon sagittal thickness (longitudinal probe) = 3.2 mm ↔

*MCL Proximal = 3.6 – 3.8 mm

*MCL Distal = 2.0 – 2.3 mm

*Tibialis Anterior Tendon (transverse probe) = 8.2 mm

*Tibialis Posterior Tendon (transverse probe) = 8.4 mm ↔

*Peroneous Longus Tendon (transverse probe) = 6.0 mm ↔

*Peroneous Brevis Tendon (transverse probe) = 4.3 mm ↔

*Achilles Tendon _A-P_ Cross-section = 5.5 – 6.5 mm ↔

*Achilles Tendon _Coronal_ = 9 – 13mm ↕

*Most tears occurs 6-7 cm proximal from attachment

*Retrocalcaneal Bursa Longitudinal length = 5.5 mm

*Retrocalcaneal Bursa (transverse probe) = 1.3 mm ↔

*Plantar Fascia thickness = 3.5 – 4.0 mm ↕

*Morton 's Neuroma = 5-7 mm diameter

THE SHOULDER

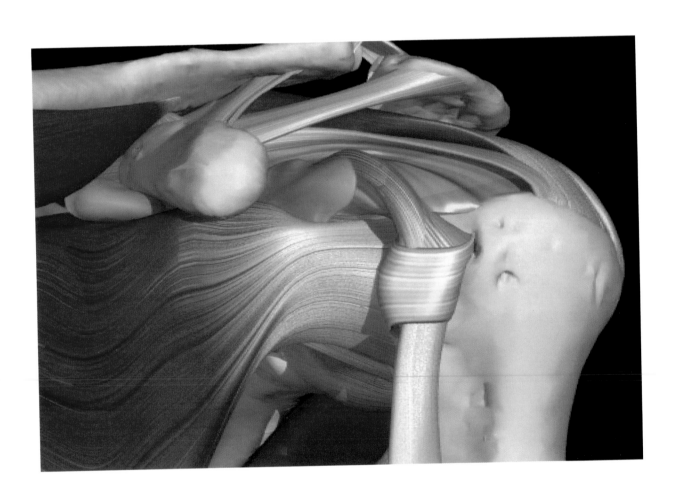

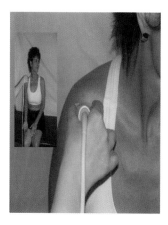

Fig. 1 Patient and probe position

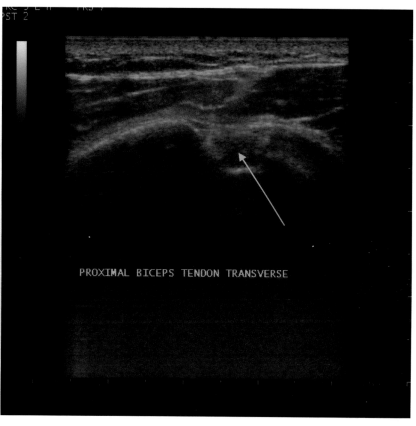

PROXIMAL BICEPS TENDON TRANSVERSE

Fig. 3: Proximal

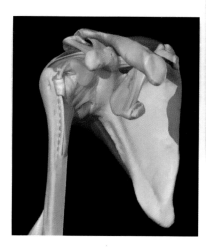

Fig. 2

The biceps tendon is imaged in both the proximal and distal regions.

Patient positioning is seated with the arm resting close to the side, and the elbow is bent at 90 degrees, resting on the patient's lap. The palm is turned up; but not actively. Sometimes a pillow is helpful when placed on the patient's lap.

Place the mid portion of the probe in transverse orientation over the PROXIMAL biceps region. By carefully aiming the sound beam the bright/echogenic contour of the humeral head will become visible.

Visualize the tendon within the bicipital groove.

LABELING: BIC PROX

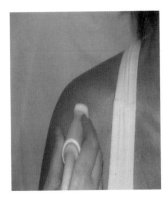

Fig. 1 Patient and probe position

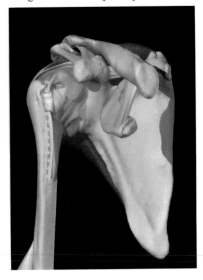

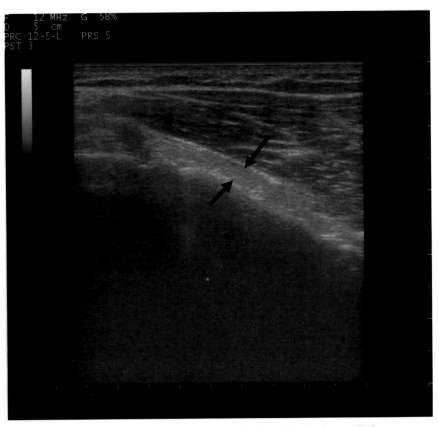

Fig. 4: Longitudinal view. Colorization applied.

1. The biceps tendon is examined in the longitudinal orientation .
   Patient positioning is unchanged (seated with the arm relaxed and the elbow flexed).

2. From the proximal transverse position, rotate the probe 90 degrees. Be careful not to let the probe slide downward. Align the probe with the long axis of the humerus.

3. The proximal biceps tendon is the hyperechoic horizontal area under the mixed echoes of the deltoid muscle.

4. To image the distal biceps tendon, simply slide the probe down approximately <u>one or two inches</u>. The tendon is seen merging into the biceps muscle.

LABELING: BIC LONG

SUBSCAPULARIS TENDON:
TRANSVERSE with EXTERNAL ROTATION

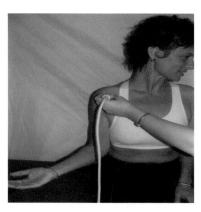

Fig. 1 Patient and probe position

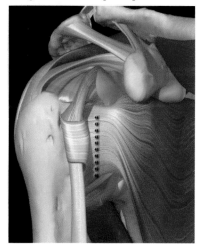

Fig. 2 : Arrows indicate
Subscapularis tendon

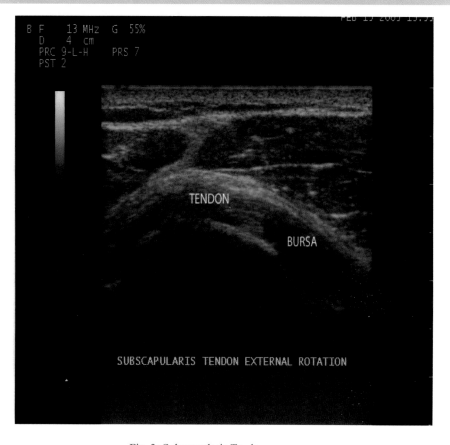

Fig. 3: Subscapularis Tendon

1. The patient is still seated with the elbow held closely to the side and bent at 90 degrees.

2. Position the probe as in the proximal biceps tendon transverse view, and slide it inferior and medially approximately one to two inches. The bicipital groove is no longer visible, but the humeral head remains in view.

3. Instruct the patient to **slowly** externally rotate the arm while keeping the elbow close to their side. The subscapularis tendon is seen gliding from the right side of the image as a horizontal echogenicity, as it attaches to the lesser tuberosity of the humerus on the left side of the image.

4. The image above demonstrates a dark area to the right of the echogenic subscapularis tendon. It is the subscapularis bursa (extending above and anterior to the tendon) being pulled laterally with the tendon during external rotation. This is not a normal image.

LABELING: SSCp TRANS EXT

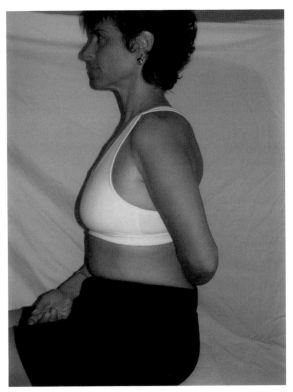

Anterior Cuff Patient Position
Supraspinatus

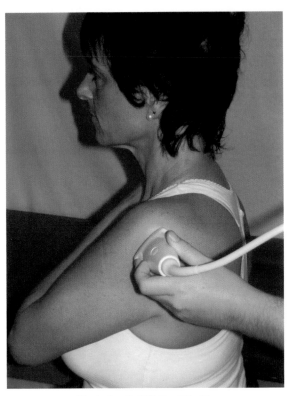

Posterior Cuff Patient Position
Infraspinatus, Teres Minor

Patient positioning is important to properly evaluate the anterior rotator cuff. It requires:
a. Full internal rotation.
b. Full posterior extension.
c. Elbow closely approximated to body.

In most cases asking the patient to rest their hand inside the back of their trousers will provide proper position and adequate patient comfort.

If proper positioning is unobtainable due to pain or restricted mobility: With the arm in a neutral position at the side, have the patient internally rotate the arm to their tolerance.

YOU SHOULD MAKE NOTE OF THE ALTERED POSITIONING ON THE IMAGES OR IN THE PATIENT FILE.

Patient positioning to evaluate the posterior cuff requires:
a. Full internal rotation.
b. Mild flexion.
c. Adduction

Asking the patient to rest their hand on the opposite shoulder will provide proper position and adequate patient comfort.

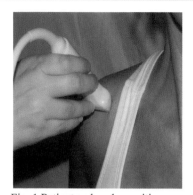

Fig. 1 Patient and probe position

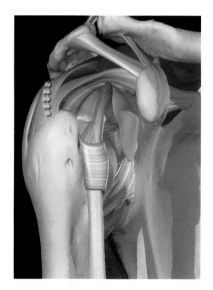

Fig. 2 Arrows indicate
Supraspinatus tendon

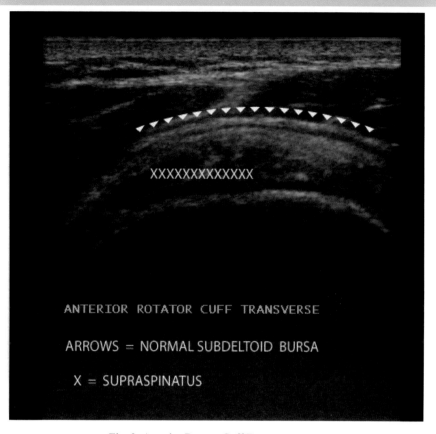

XXXXXXXXXXXXX

ANTERIOR ROTATOR CUFF TRANSVERSE

ARROWS = NORMAL SUBDELTOID BURSA

X = SUPRASPINATUS

Fig. 3: Anterior Rotator Cuff Transverse

1. Place the probe in the anterior transverse orientation at approximately the mid portion of the gleno-humeral joint.

2. The thick/wide, bright/echogenic arc is the supraspinatus tendon.

3. The thin/slender, dark/anechoic area just above the tendon is the synovial lining of the subdeltoid/ subacromial bursa in its normal state.
Normally; the bursa is small, with a flat echogenic lining. Bursal effusion is many times secondary to tendon degeneration.

LABELING: SSP TRANS

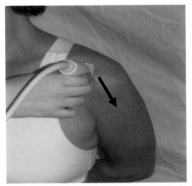

Fig. 1 Probe parallel to Humeral shaft

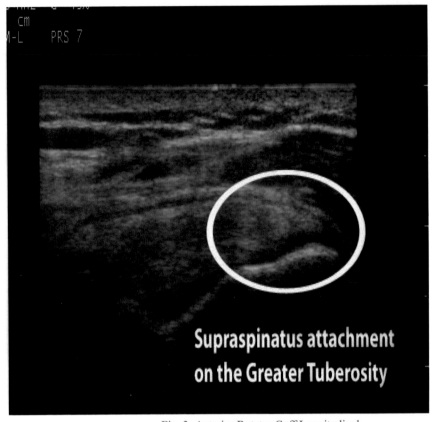

Supraspinatus attachment
on the Greater Tuberosity

Fig. 3: Anterior Rotator Cuff Longitudinal

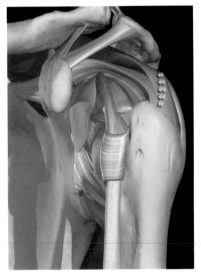

Fig. 2 Arrows indicate
Supraspinatus tendon

1. From the anterior transverse position, ROTATE THE PROBE 90 DEGREES.
   On longitudinal views, the left side of the monitor is toward the patient's head.

2. Viewing the image from right to left, the supraspinatus tendon resembles a "birds beak". The point of the beak is the insertion of the tendon onto the greater tuberosity of the humerus.

3. The anechoic/black area on the articular surface is the tendon footprint, which is normal.

* The "Critical Zone" is the 1 cm avascular area at the lateral margin of the supraspinatus tendon, where 90 % of all rotator cuff tears are found.

   LABELING: SSP LONG

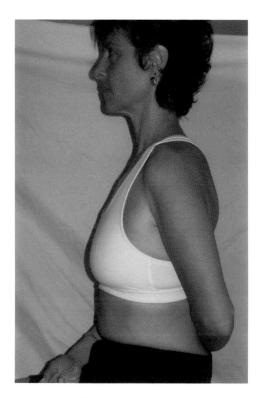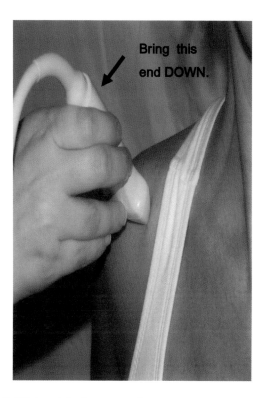

Bring this
end DOWN.

Fig. 1 and 2 : Patient and probe position for the Rotator Cuff Interval is the same as the
Anterior SSP image. WITH SUPERIOR to INFERIOR probe angle.

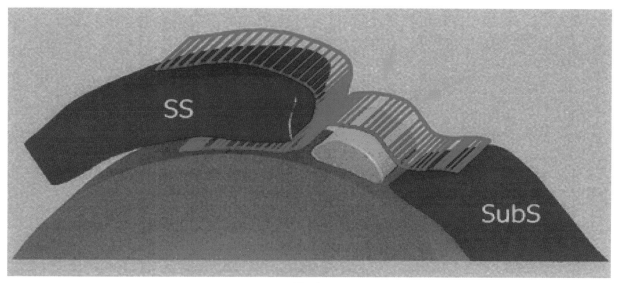

SS

SubS

Fig. 3
The Biceps tendon enters the Gleno-Humeral joint through the
Rotator Cuff Interval

RC Interval image on following page.

ROTATOR CUFF INTERVAL
Evaluate for Adhesive Capsulitis

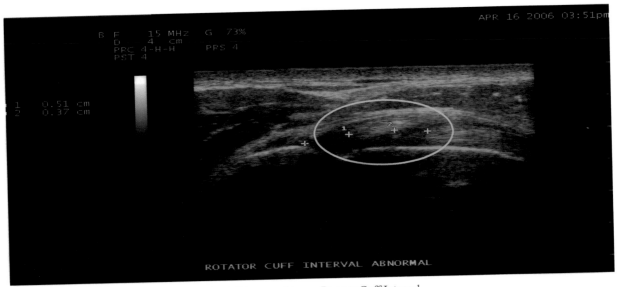

Fig. 1 Ultrasound image Rotator Cuff Interval

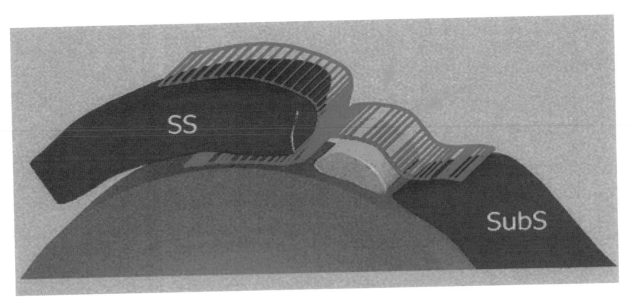

Fig. 2 Diagram Rotator Cuff Interval

1. The normal interval (SSP and/or SSC) is 3mm or less. Measurements greater than 3mm are indicative of adhesive capsulitis or fluid in the tendon sheath.

2. The joint capsule s deep to BT. Effusion increases interval between the SSP and SSC

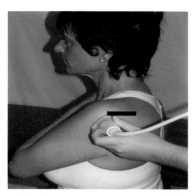

Fig. 1 Transverse probe position

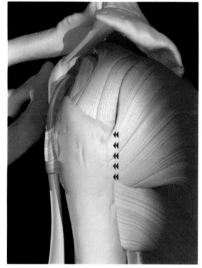

Fig. 2: Infraspinatus in yellow.
Attachment at arrows.

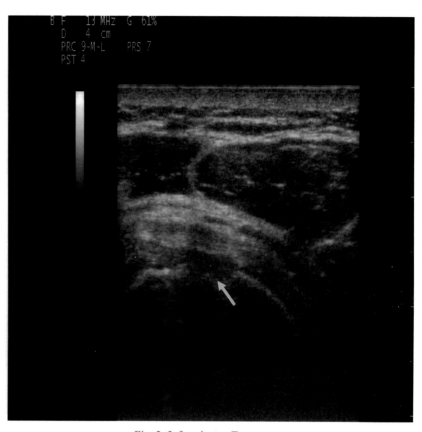

Fig. 3: Infraspinatus Transverse
Arrow indicates a common anatomic variant that is often accentuated in
throwing athletes and swimmers.

1. From the Supraspinatus transverse position, slide the probe laterally to a position that is slightly posterior /oblique on the shoulder. The humeral head outline remains visible. The fibers of the infraspinatus tendon will be seen. A notch is commonly seen in the humerus deep to the musculo-tendinous junction. This is a normal finding, and may be accentuated in throwing athletes.

2. Visualize the bright/echogenic arc the infraspinatus tendon. The thin/slender, dark area just above the tendon is the subdeltoid/subacromial bursa in its normal state. See SSP transverse page. Normally; the bursa is small, with a flat echogenic lining. Bursal effusion is many times secondary to tendon degeneration.

LABELING: Inf Sp TRANS

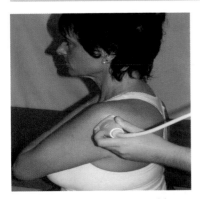

Fig. 1 Longitudinal probe position

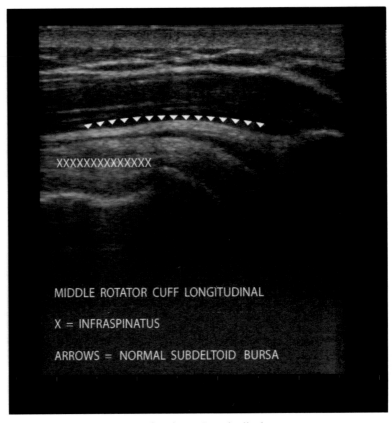

MIDDLE ROTATOR CUFF LONGITUDINAL

X = INFRASPINATUS

ARROWS = NORMAL SUBDELTOID BURSA

Fig. 3: Infraspinatus Longitudinal

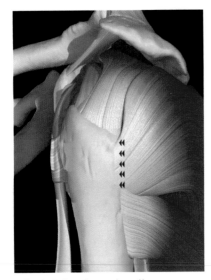

Fig. 2: Infraspinatus in yellow.
Attachment at arrows.

1. From the Infraspinatus transverse position, ROTATE THE PROBE 90 DEGREES.

2. By viewing from right to left, the cuff still resembles a "birds beak" except it is flattened or more wedge-like. This is the broad attachment of infraspinatus tendon. The thin, anechoic/dark area just above the tendon is the subdeltoid/subacromial bursa in its normal state.

3. The outline of the humeral head is visible. When both the rotator cuff tendon, and the humeral head are seen; freeze the image.

   LABELING: Inf Sp LONG

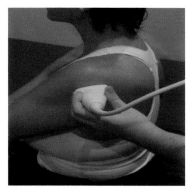

Fig. 1 Probe is inferior to Inf Sp.

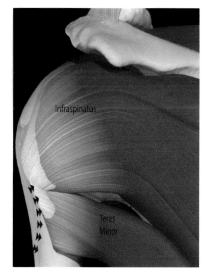

Fig. 2: Teres minor in yellow and marked by arrows.

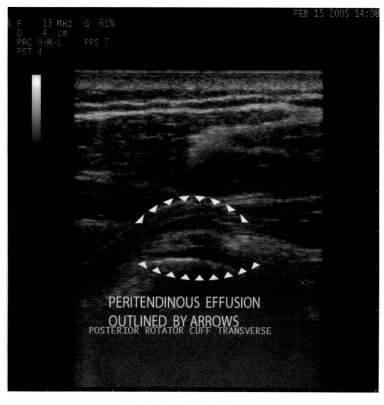

PERITENDINOUS EFFUSION
OUTLINED BY ARROWS
POSTERIOR ROTATOR CUFF TRANSVERSE

Fig. 3: Teres Minor Transverse
Rare Teres Minor peri-tendon effusion seen above

1. Slide the probe inferiorly from the infraspinatus tendon position. The probe will still be in an oblique position to the long axis of the humerus, as in the infraspinatus images.

2. Visualize the echogenic arc of the teres minor just above the humeral head. Due to the inferior position required to scan the teres minor tendon, the humeral head may be somewhat difficult to see.

3. The image above demonstrates peritendinous effusion above and below the teres minor tendon. The Teres Minor is rarely pathologic, and rarely imaged on routine shoulder exams.

LABELING: TM TRANS

ROTATOR CUFF:
Teres Minor Longitudinal View

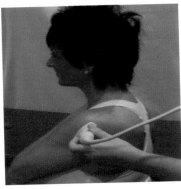
Fig. 1 Long axis BELOW Inf Sp

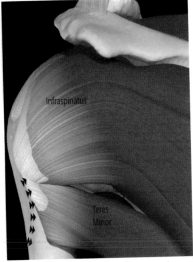
Fig. 2: Teres minor in yellow and marked by arrows.

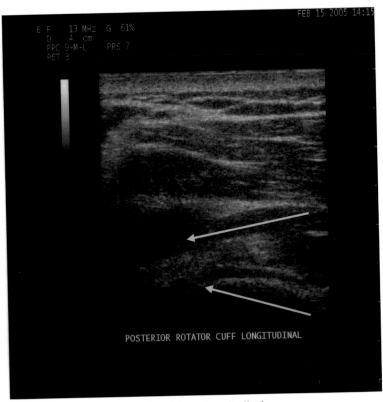
Fig. 3: Teres Minor Longitudinal
Reading right to left; the TM narrows to it's Greater Tuberosity attachment

1. From the TM transverse position, ROTATE THE PROBE 90 DEGREES. The left side of the monitor is cephalad.

2. Scanning from the posterior will continue to flatten the "birds beak" appearance of the rotator cuff tendons.
   Reading from right to left; the Teres Minor muscle narrows to its tendon attachment on the Greater Tuberosity.

LABELING: TM LONG

ACROMIO-CLAVICULAR JOINT

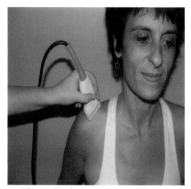

Fig. 1: Probe position: Obliquely
transverse across AC joint

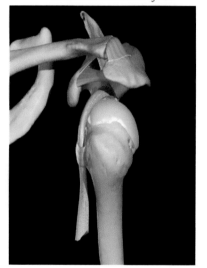

Fig. 2 Acromio-clavicular ligament
in yellow.

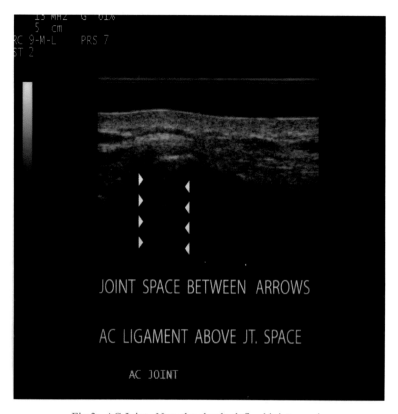

JOINT SPACE BETWEEN ARROWS

AC LIGAMENT ABOVE JT. SPACE

AC JOINT

Fig 3: AC Joint . Note the clearly defined joint margin

1. The patient is seated. <u>Instruct them to sit up quite straight while relaxing the shoulders.</u>

2. Place the probe obliquely transverse across the AC joint, near the most lateral portion of the clavicle.

3. Two (2) separate black bony shadows will be identified.
   The <u>left</u> shadow is the <u>acromion</u> of the scapula.
   The <u>right</u> shadow is lateral/distal <u>clavicle.</u> The clavicle is usually abit superior to the acromion.

4. Measure the joint space between the acromion and the clavicle using internal calipers of the scanner.
   Measure "Edge to Edge". From the <u>medial edge</u> of the acromion on the left.
   to the <u>lateral edge</u> of the clavicle on the right. This provides measurement of the visible joint space, and not the bony landmarks.
   LABELING: LT AC or RT AC

ACROMIO-CLAVICULAR JOINT
Measurement for Shoulder Separation

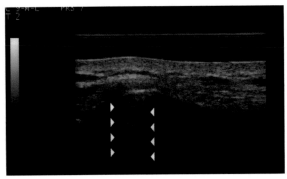

Fig. 1: Grayscale AC image

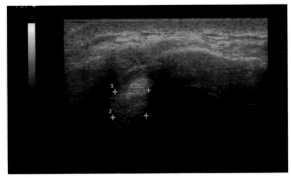

Fig 2: Colorized image more clearly defines joint margin

Tossy Calculated Index For Shoulder Separation

Normal/Asymptomatic side measurement

DIVIDED BY

Abnormal/Symptomatic side measurement

Class I = 1.0 +/- Basic sprain of ligaments

Class II = 0.49- 0.50 +/-Partial tear

Class III = 0.21 +/- Complete rupture

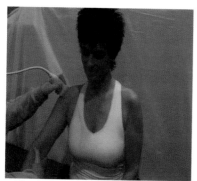

Fig. 1: Longitudinal probe position.
Oblique to see Acr and Humerus

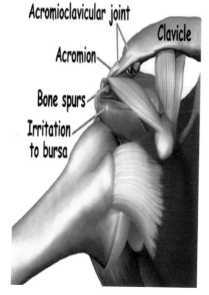

Fig. 2 : Flexion with Abduction
abuts the SSP against the Acr

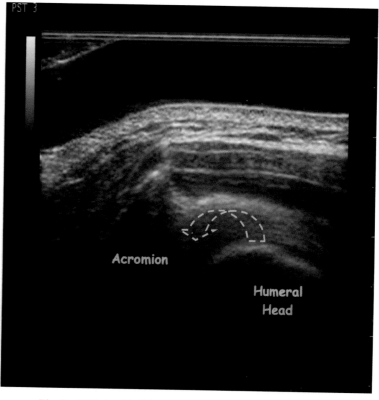

Fig. 3 : SSP should slide unobstructed under the Acromion with
Humeral flexion and Abduction.

1. Dynamic imaging is required to determine shoulder impingement.
2. Place the probe in a longitudinal-oblique orientation high enough on the humerus to visualize the boney landmarks of the Acromion and the Humeral Head.
3. Maintain probe contact as <u>the examiner</u> SLOWLY raises the patient arm in flexion-Abduction
4. The Supraspinatus tendon should slide smoothly from right to left, and disappear under the Acromion.

LABELING : Shldr Imp

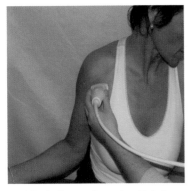

Fig 1 External rotation. Inferior
probe position at the axilla.

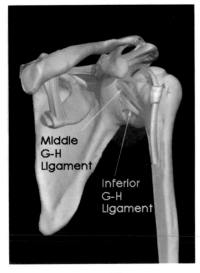

Fig 2 Gleno-Humeral ligaments are
superficial to the Labrum

Middle
G-H
Ligament

Inferior
G-H
Ligament

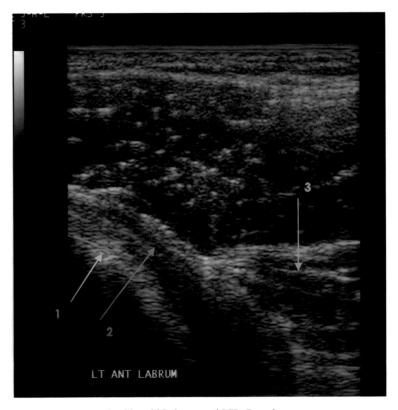

LT ANT LABRUM

1= Glenoid Labrum and IGL Complex
2= Gleno-Humeral Capsule
3= Subscapularis Muscle

1. The patient is seated with the elbow held closely to the side, flexed at 90 degrees with external
   rotation to expose the anterior glenoid labrum.

2. Position the probe in a transverse orientation, and slide it inferior and medially toward the axilla.

3. Identify the boney landmark of the humeral head . The middle and inferior gleno-humeral
   Ligament complex ,and the anterior glenoid labrum can be difficult to distinguish separately.

4. Anterior instability due to Inferior G-H ligament laxity or disruption is common.
    Bankart's Lesion is an avulsion of the IGH ligament *from* the labrum.
    Ultrasound has limited access to the labrum.

LABELING: ANT GH LAB

GLENOID LABRUM : Posterior

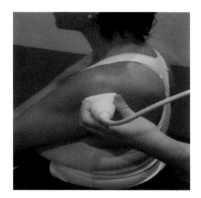

Patient Position: Internal rotation
with adduction

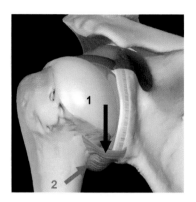

1= Inf. G H Ligament
2= Axillary Pouch of GHL

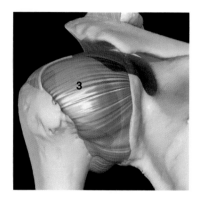

Note SUPERIOR location of Joint
Capsule (3) relative to IGL

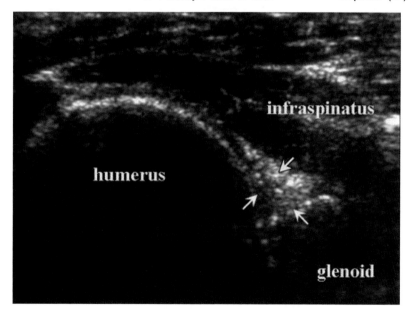

1. The patient is seated with the upper extremity in full adduction and internal rotation to expose the posterior gleno-humeral joint and labrum.

2. Position the probe in a transverse orientation, and slide it inferior and medially into the axilla. Probe position high on the shoulder will visualize the capsule, and not the labrum.

3. Inferior to superior probe angle with adequate probe pressure is necessary to visualize the peripheral margin of the labrum.

LABELING: POST GH LAB

THE ELBOW

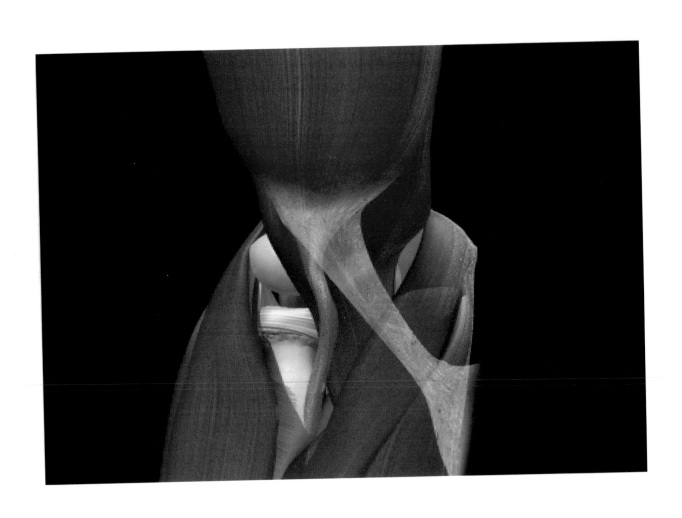

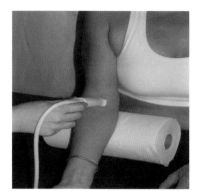

Fig. 1 Transverse probe with full extention of elbow

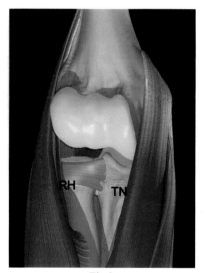

Fig 2

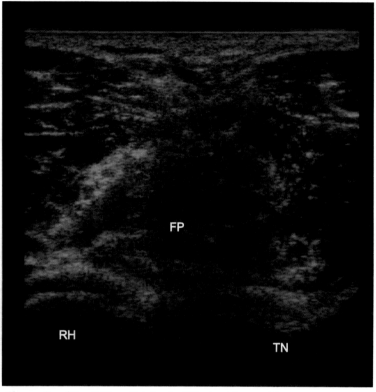

Figures 2 and 3 : RH= radial head   TN = trochlear notch
FP = anterior fat pad

1. Place probe transversely on the elbow at the level of, <u>or just slightly below</u> the antecubital fossa.

2. The radio-ulnar joint is visualized. A small "crescent shaped" echogenicity on the left is the radial head. The bright, concave cortical outline of the trochlear notch is on the right.
The extensor muscles are above and left of the radial head. The forearm flexor muscles are on the right side of the image.

3. Anterior compartment effusions will displace the anterior fat pad.

LABELING: ANT TRANS ELB

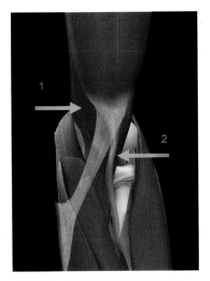

Fig. 1 Brachialis MUSCLE (1) is <u>deep</u>
to Biceps TENDON (2)

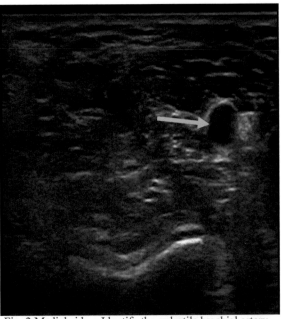

Fig. 2 Medial side : Identify the pulsatile brachial artery.

1. Probe orientation and patient position are the
    same as previous image.

2. To recognize the biceps tendon, first move the
   probe to the medial side of the fossa. Identify the
   pulsatile brachial artery. The median nerve may
   also be seen adjacent to the artery.Fig 2.

3. Moving the probe in a lateral direction toward midline, the biceps tendon will be seen centrally
   Located, and on top of the brachialis muscle.
   The tendon will likely appear dark/hypoechoic due
   to anisotropy. Fig. 3

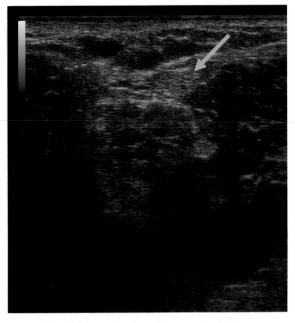

Fig. 1 Move probe laterally toward midline.
Biceps tendon is seen as a hypoechoic oval near
top

NOTE: The distal biceps tendon does not have
       a tendon sheath, and therefore cannot
       develop tenosynvitis.

DISTAL BICEPS TENDON
Longitudinal (radial tuberosity attachment)

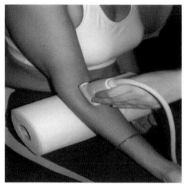

Fig. 1 Longitudinal probe position.
Slight LATERAL beam angle

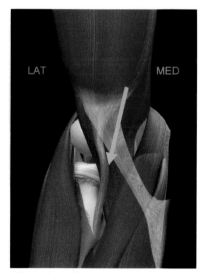

Fig.2 Lateral beam angle
Helps with BT visualization

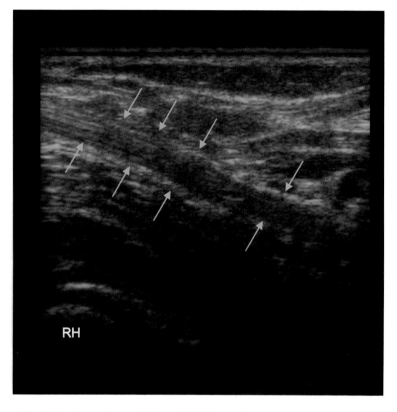

Fig 3 The dense, hyperechoic and fibrillar tendon takes an oblique course to the radial tuberosity attachment. RH= radial head

1. Probe is in longitudinal orientation with a slight LATERAL beam angle to ensure imaging of the biceps tendon, and not the medially located brachialis tendon .The patient 's arm remains fully extended.

2. Applying significant probe pressure, and using " h eel-toe " maneuvering helps to track the biceps tendon to the radial tuberosity. The oblique course the tendon follows makes it difficult to trace.

LABELING: DIS BT LONG

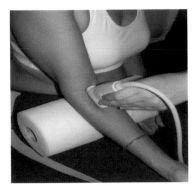

Fig. 1 Longitudinal probe position.
Slight MEDIAL beam angle

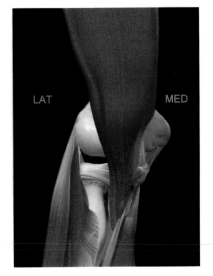

Fig.2 Medial beam angle
to see Brachialis tendon

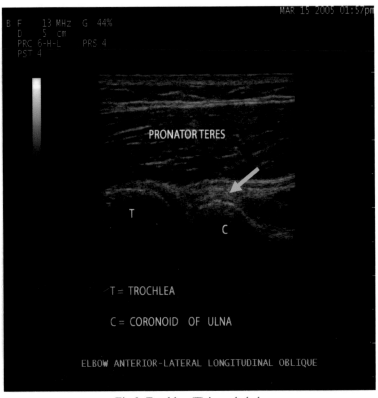

Fig 3 Trochlea (T) is cephalad.
Coronoid (C) is caudal
Brachialis tendon (1) is deep to Pronator Teres

1. Probe is in longitudinal orientation with a slight MEDIAL beam angle to ensure imaging of the BRACHIALIS tendon, and not the LATERALLY positioned biceps tendon .The patient 's arm remains fully extended.

2. Identify the boney landmarks of the humeral trochlea (T) , and the ulnar Coronoid   (C) .

3. The Brachialis tendon attaches on the on the anterior surface of the Coronoid .
    LABELING: BRK TEN LONG

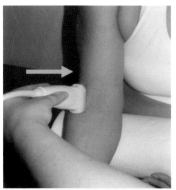

Fig. 1 Longitudinal probe position
on lateral aspect <u>and</u> superior
at the epicondyle .

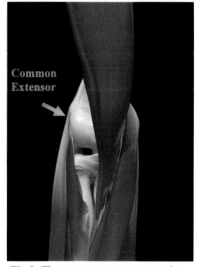

**Common
Extensor**

Fig.2 The common extensor attaches
superior/proximal to capitellum

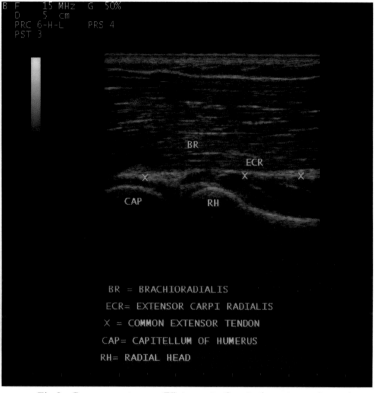

Fig 3   Common extensor (X) tapers to the attachment superior to the
capitellum.

1.   Position the probe out on the lateral aspect of the elbow in a longitudinal plane.
     The boney landmarks are the capitellum of the humerus (proximal) ,and the radial head (distal)

2. Just above the capitellum is the insertion of the common forearm extensor tendon,
    superior to the lateral epicondyle. The extensor muscles are to the right and above
    the extensor tendon. (radialis brevis and longus, extensor radialis).

LABELING: LAT EPI LONG

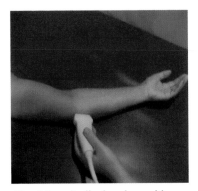

Fig. 1 Longitudinal probe position on medial aspect with supination.

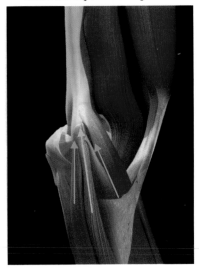

Fig.2 A direct medial to lateral view of the medial epicondyle. The common flexor (yellow) and flexor superficialis (green) converge on the condyle.

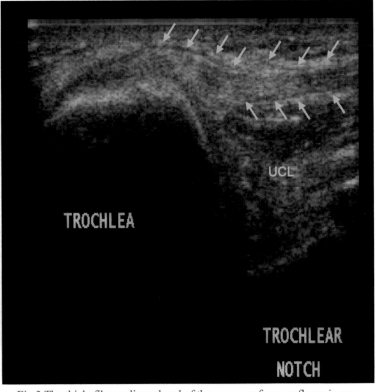

UCL

TROCHLEA

TROCHLEAR

NOTCH

Fig 3 The thick, fibrous linear band of the common forearm flexor is seen superficial the ulnar collateral ligament.

1. The elbow remains fully extended. <u>The hand is actively supinated</u>. Ask the patient to turn the palm upward.

2. Place the probe in a longitudinal plane on the medial side of the elbow. The probe is parallel with the forearm. The ulno humeral joint is seen. The boney landmark on the right of the image is the trochlear notch of the ulna. Just to the left is the echogenic arc of the humeral trochlea. The pronator teres over- lies the trochlea, and may be seen as over-lying the common flexor tendon.

3. The common flexor tendon and the flexor superficialis converge to attach on the condyle.

LABELING: MED EPI LONG

ULNAR NERVE IMAGING
Cross-sectional area measurement

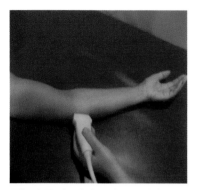

Fig. 1 Probe below the condyle.
Obliquely crossing ulnar groove.

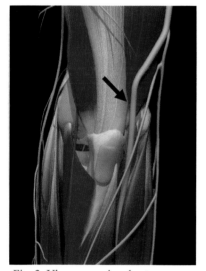

Fig. 2 Ulnar nerve is subcutaneous
and within the ulnar groove.

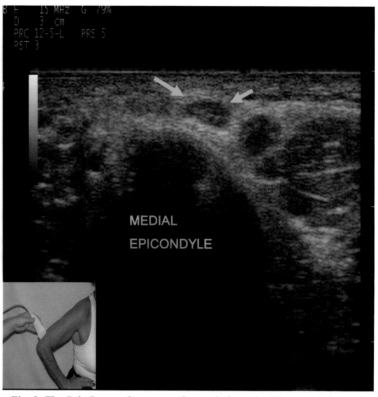

MEDIAL
EPICONDYLE

Fig. 3 The Sub-Q nerve is seen as a hypoechoic <u>oval</u> with punctate internal
foci ,characteristic of a peripheral nerve, adjacent to the medial
epicondyle. The rounded, dark structure next to the nerve is FCU muscle.

1. This image can be performed with the elbow extended, or in the "crab" position. See inset fig. 3.

2. On the extended elbow, place the probe just "below" the condyle, and crossing the ulnar groove.
   The cortical outline of the medial epicondyle is the boney landmark.

3. The subcutaneous ulnar nerve is a hypoechoic _ovoid_ structure with punctate internal foci adjacent to the condyle. The round, dark structure next to the nerve is the flexor carpi ulnaris muscle.

4. Cross-sectional measurement : 7.5 to 9.0 mm is an acceptable range thought to be "normal".
   Varied opinions exist. Bilateral measurements are recommended as nerve swelling is
   considered good criteria for entrapment.

LABELING: ULN NRV X-SEC

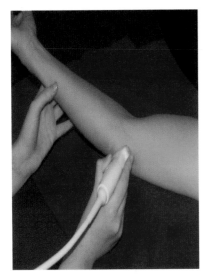

Fig. 1 Extended elbow
Obliquely crossing ulnar groove.

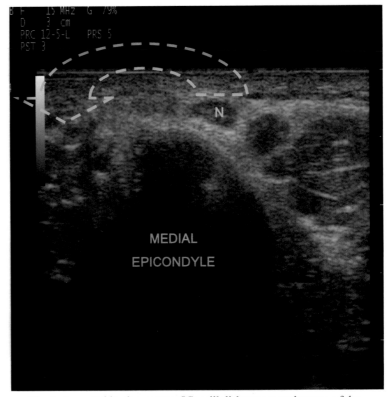

MEDIAL

EPICONDYLE

Fig. 3 An unstable ulnar nerve (N), will dislocate over the apex of the
medial epicondyle with elbow flexion.

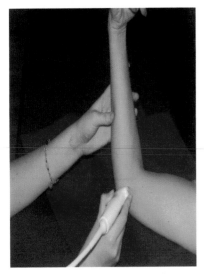

Fig. 2 Flexed elbow
Maintain probe contact during flexion.

1. On the extended elbow, place the probe just "below" the condyle, and crossing the ulnar groove. The cortical outline of the medial epicondyle is the boney landmark.

2. The subcutaneous ulnar nerve is a hypoechoic *ovoid* structure with punctate internal foci .

3. The examiner slowly flexes the elbow, maintaining full probe contact ,and watching the nerve to observe movement over the apex of the medial epicondyle.

LABELING : ULN NRV SUBLUX

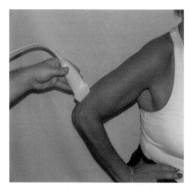

Fig. 1 Longitudinal probe position.
Patient in "Crab" position.

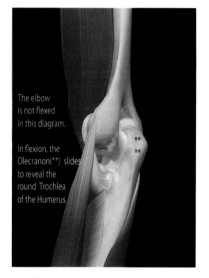

The elbow is not flexed in this diagram.

In flexion, the Olecranon(**) slides to reveal the round Trochlea of the Humerus

Fig.2 Triceps tendon and muscle not shown.

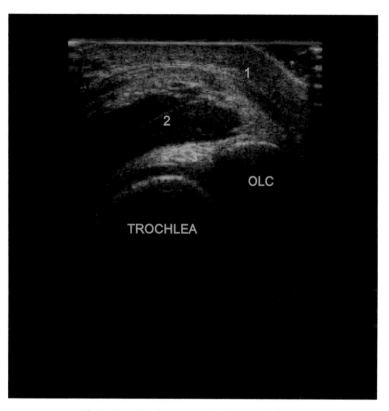

Fig.3 Trochlea is proximal. Olecranon is distal.
1 = Superficial triceps tendon
2 = Triceps muscle
3 = Posterior joint capsule

1. By asking the patient to rest his/her palm on their hip, proper positioning is obtained to scan the posterior aspect of the elbow (elevation, flexion, abduction). AKA the "crab" position.

2. The probe is placed on the posterior elbow, parallel with the long axis of the humerus.

3. The trochlea of the humerus is a round bony landmark at the left portion of the screen. The posterior joint capsule is a diagonal hyperechoic strip on top of the trochlea. The triceps brachii muscle is above the capsule.

4. At the top of the image, the tendon of the triceps is seen as a bright linear band. The triceps tendon is seen above the muscle.

LABELING: POST ELB LONG

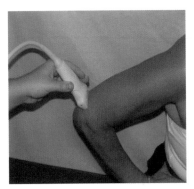

Fig. 1 Transverse probe position.
Patient in "Crab" position.

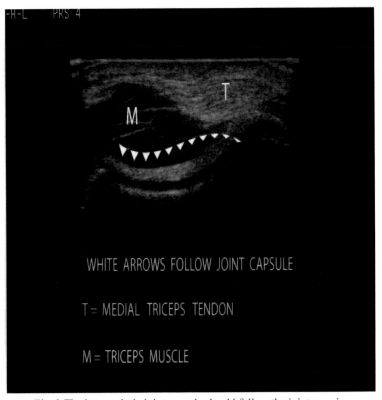

WHITE ARROWS FOLLOW JOINT CAPSULE

T = MEDIAL TRICEPS TENDON

M = TRICEPS MUSCLE

Fig. 3 The hyperechoic joint capsule should follow the joint margin.
Fluid accumulations will displace the capsule upward.

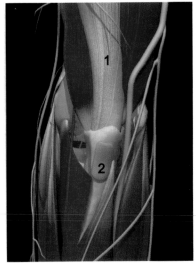

Fig. 2 Note the superficial portion of
the triceps tendon (1) ,with muscle
deep to it. The OLC bursa (2) will be
moved distally in elbow flexion.

1. The patient remains in the"crab" position as in the longitudinal view (elevation, flexion,
   and abduction).

3. The joint margin should be well defined.
   A bright horizontal echogenicity is the fibrous posterior joint capsule. The triceps brachii
   is above the capsule.   The medial portion of the triceps tendon is seen above and right to the
   muscle on the image above.

LABELING: POST ELB TRANS

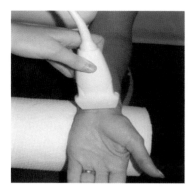

Fig. 1 Supported wrist
Neutral position

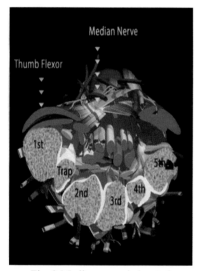

Fig. 2 Median nerve is located
toward the Radial aspect, not true
midline.

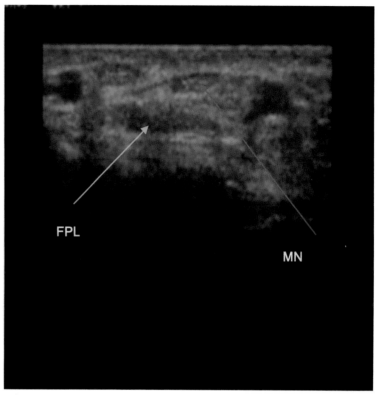

Fig. 3 Ask patient to flex the thumb. Median nerve (MN) is above and right of
the flexor pollicis (FPL). Visualize bright, punctuate foci of nerve fibers.

1. The patient's wrist is in a neutral position with the palm up. Using a pillow allows the wrist to be relaxed, and eliminates any flexion or extension.

2. Place the probe transversely across the wrist at the flexor retinaculum.

3. The flexor tendons are in compartments. They appear as echogenic ovoid structures on transverse examination. Unfortunately; so does the median nerve.

4. The median nerve is superficial to the flexor pollicis longus tendon, and distinguishable from the flexor tendons by identifying it's punctuate or pinpoint internal echoes.

5. Slowly flex the thumb, and look for tendon movement. The median nerve will be stationary.

LABELING: PAL TRANS

MEDIAN NERVE CROSS-SECTIONAL MEASUREMENT

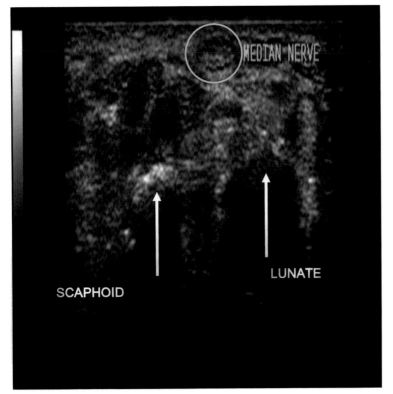

Fig. 1 Identify the hypoechoic,ovoid median nerve, with characteristic
punctate internal foci.
Boney landmarks on the right wrist are Scaphoid and Lunate.

Fig 2 Cross sectional measurement
of median nerve

1. Locate the median nerve as a hypoechoic, ovoid structure with the characteristic punctuate internal foci demonstrated by peripheral nerves in short axis. On a right wrist, the
boney landmarks are the scaphoid on the left, and lunate on the right.

2. Most ultrasound scanners have either an "ellipse" or "trace" measurement feature that
will produce a cross-sectional area measurement.

3. Currently accepted ranges of normal median nerve cross-sectional area:

Normal (male) = 7-9 mm

Normal (female) = 5-7mm

Greater than 9mm (male/female) = abnormal

Split-screen function allows comparative views

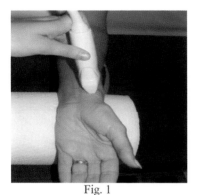

Fig. 1

1. The probe is longitudinal, off–midline to the radial margin. Fig 1

2. The palmaris longus is superficial to the median nerve. Reading the image from top to bottom, the palmaris longus, PL, is first, then the median nerve, MN. *Hyperechoic* superficial flexor tendons ,SF, are deep to the nerve, followed by *hypoechoic* muscle of the deep flexors, DF. Fig 2 & 3

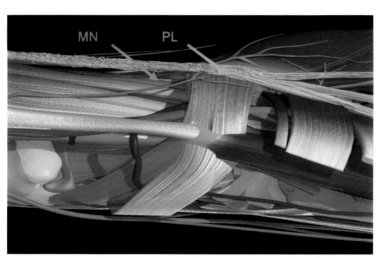

Fig. 2

Scan Tip:

On dynamic imaging, the palmaris longus is not a sliding tendon, like the other flexor tendons. It's function is to tense the skin of the palm while gripping.

Slowly flexing the fingers will demonstrate the sliding motion of the flexor tendons. The nerve is stationary.

REMEMBER: Peripheral nerves on long axis are distinguishable from tendons by noting…

" Parallel hyperechoic lines with dark separations. "

Inflammation of the median nerve will give it a fusiform shape. A normal nerve has a uniform " ribbon-like " appearance.

LABELING: PAL LONG

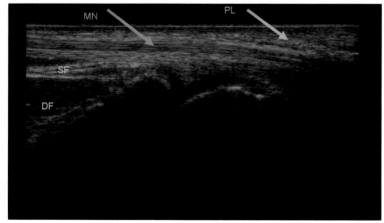

Fig. 3
Dynamic imaging shows sliding flexors and stationary median nerve.

THE WRIST and HAND

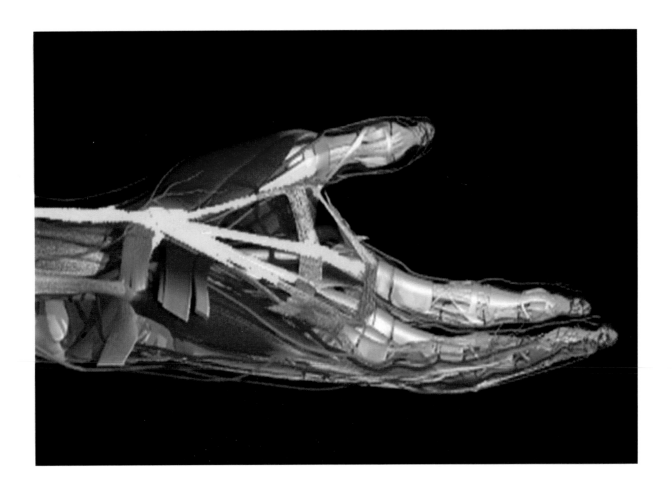

DORSAL TRANSVERSE WRIST

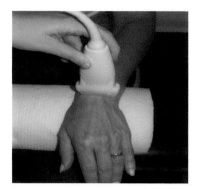

Fig. 1 Transverse probe over the extensor retinaculum

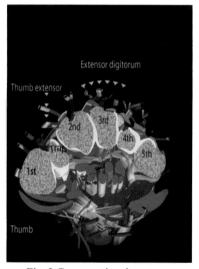

Fig. 2 Cross-sectional anatomy

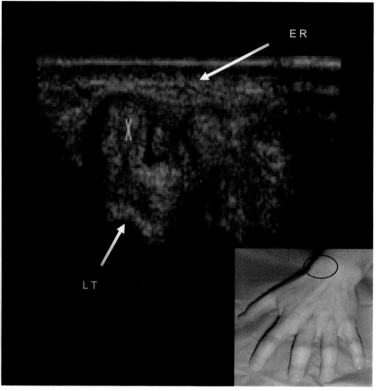

Fig. 3 Extensor Pollicis Longus (X) is the largest tendon of the three radial extensor compartments, deep to the extensor retinaculum (ER). Lister's tubercle (LT) is the boney landmark. Note arrow and inset photo

1. The patient's wrist is in a neutral position with the palm down.

2. The probe is placed transversely across the wrist, over the extensor retinaculum.

3. Lister's tubercle ,of the distal radius, is the most prominent boney landmark on the dorsal wrist. The extensor pollicis longus tendon wraps around Lister's tubercle ,on the ulnar side of the tubercle.

4. The extensor tendons are in compartments beneath the retinaculum. The three compartments on the radial side are usually more visible. The largest tendon is the extensor pollicis longus of the thumb.

5. Extension and abduction of the thumb allows visualization of the EPL from the tubercle to the base of the thumb phalanx. In rheumatoid arthritis , pathology of the EPL is common.

LABELING: DOR TRANS

DORSAL LONGITUDINAL WRIST

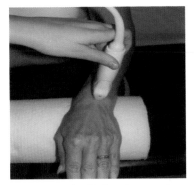

Fig. 1 Longitudinal probe over the
extensor retinaculum

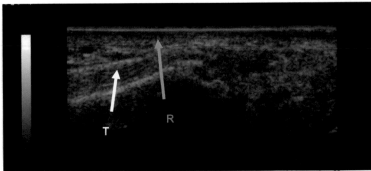

Fig. 3 Longitudinal extensor tendon image. No acoustic stand-off.
T = tendon   R = retinaculum

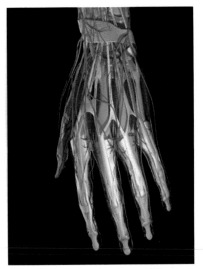

Fig. 2 Surface anatomy of the
dorsal wrist

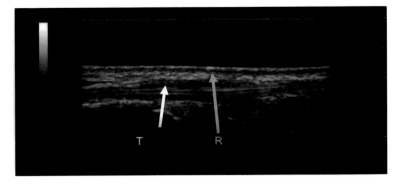

Fig. 4 Longitudinal extensor tendon image. Acoustic stand-off employed.

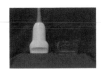

1. The wrist is in a neutral position with no flexion or extension. Place the probe in
   the longitudinal plane.

2. The extensor tendons are the bright echogenic bands just beneath the extensor retinaculum.
   There are six (6) extensor tendon compartments. This example simply demonstrates a general
   mid-line probe placement, and sample image of an extensor tendon in long axis view.

   The examiner must determine specific tendon compartments to visualize based on clinical
   presentation.

3. Note the difference in distinguishing the tendon (T) from the overlying retinaculum (R)
   by using an acoustic stand-off on the images above (Figs. 3 and 4). Acoustic stand-offs are
   beneficial in visualizing superficial structures passing over and near boney prominences.

LABELING: DOR LONG (1st thru 6th)

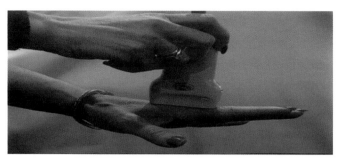

Fig. 1 Longitudinal probe crossing the MCP joint

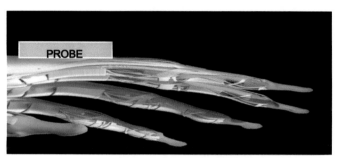

PROBE

Fig. 2 Surface anatomy of dorsal MCP

1. Place the probe in the longitudinal plane over the MCP joint of interest. The metacarpal head is rounded,and presents a significant boney prominence.

2. The extensor digitorum (ED) tendon is most superficial. Deep to the tendon are the transverse interosseous tendons (TI), and collateral ligaments. Fig 2

Both of which cross the joint space . It is difficult to distinguish them as separate structures with sonography.

3. The MCP is frequently affected in rheumatoid arthritis, as well as the PIP. Joint effusions, synovitis, soft-tissue swelling can be easily detected and monitored with ultrasound. Cortical erosions of the MCP will be plainly evident. Fig 4

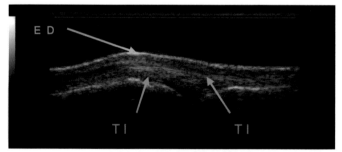

ED

TI   TI

Fig. 3 Longitudinal image of dorsal MCP.
Acoustic stand-off employed

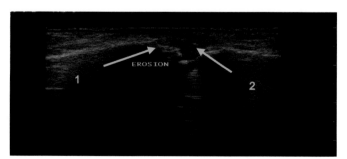

EROSION

1   2

Fig. 4 Active RA . Longitudinal image of dorsal MCP joint.
Cortical erosion (1)
No anechoic hyaline cartilage and joint effusion (2)

PALMAR METACARPAL-PHALANGEAL TRANSVERSE
The A1 Pulley

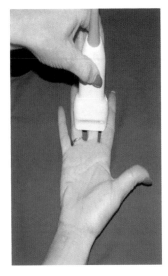

Fig. 1 Transverse probe over
the most proximal A1 pulley

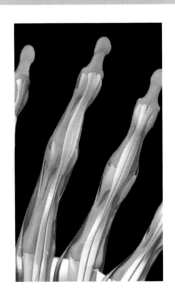

Fig. 2

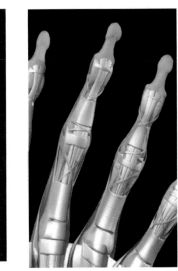

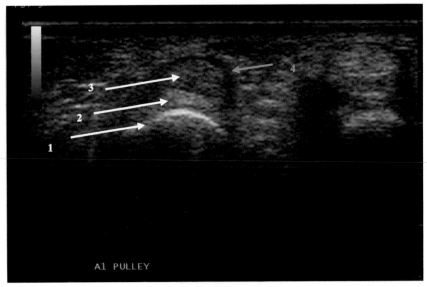

Fig. 3 **Reading from cortex up**
1= cortical outline of metacarpal head
2= volar plate
3= flexor digitorum profundus
4= A1 pulley arching over the tendon

Clinical Significance : Common site of "trigger finger". A thickened flexor or a
nodule on the tendon will catch on the pulley, causing momentary locking of the
finger in flexion.   LABELING : A1 PULL TRANS

THENAR LONGITUDINAL VIEWS
Radial Side

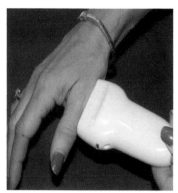

Fig. 1 Long axis probe , radial side.

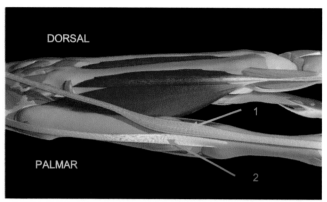

Fig. 2   Extensor pollicis longus (1)
Extensor pollicis brevis (2)

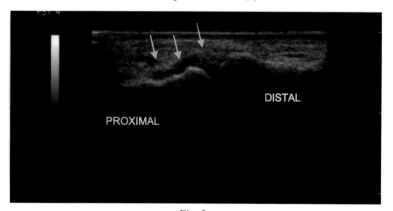

Fig. 3
EPL and EPB cross the 1st MCP joint.
There is no ligament deep to the tendons.

1.   Place the probe in a longitudinal orientation on the radial side of the thumb.

NOTE : Do not allow the probe to slip inferiorly or toward the palmar aspect.
            Lower probe placement will not visualize the extensors of the thumb.

2. The boney landmark on the left is the 1st metacarpal head. On the left is the proximal phalanx of the thumb.

3. The extensor pollicis longus and brevis both cross the metacarpal phalangeal joint. The tendons are quite thin, and closely approximated, making them difficult to visualize as separate structures. Using the base of the proximal phalanx as a landmark helps locate the attachment of the EPB.

NOTE: There is no ligament deep to the tendons.
        De Quervain's Stenosing Tenosynovitis (involving EPB and Abductor Pollicis Longus) is best seen <u>proximal to the extensor retinaculum</u>

LABELING: THUMB EXT LONG

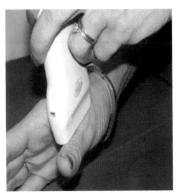

Fig.1 Long axis probe, ulnar side.
Stay medial of EPL

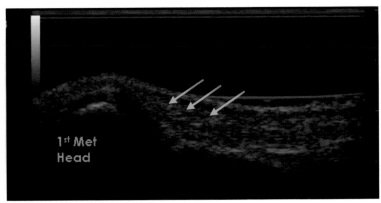

Fig.3 Collateral ligament crosses the joint space
Note anechoic rim of hyaline cartilage deep to ligament

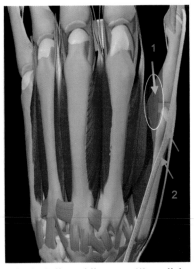

Fig. 2 Collateral ligament (1) medial
of EPL (2)

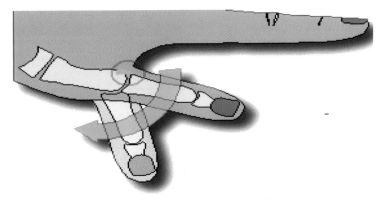

Fig.4 Falling forward and catching the thumb will hyper– Abduct the
1st MCP joint and injure the collateral ligament.

1. Place the probe in a longitudinal orientation on the ulnar side of the thumb.

NOTE : Stay medial of the EPL. Gently ABduct the patient's thumb for probe access.

2. The boney landmark on the left is the 1st metacarpal head. On the left is the proximal phalanx of the thumb.

3. The ulnar collateral ligament is the linear band crossing the MCP joint. Ligaments are characterized as not being as bright as tendons, and also not displaying such distinct fibrous texture as tendons.

4. The UCL is often torn in hyper– Abduction injuries ie. Game Keeper's and Skier's Thumb injuries. Avulsion fractures can be seen on ultrasound. Check cortical continuity of metatarsal Head.

LABELING : THUMB UCL LONG

TRIANGULAR FIBROCARTILAGE COMPLEX
TFCC

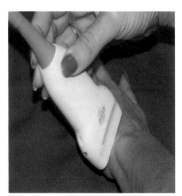

Fig.1 Oblique probe position on ulnar aspect. Pt. radial deviation

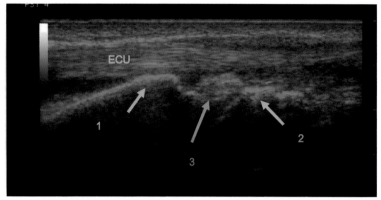

Fig.3 Maintaining a more dorsal/ulnar probe position across the ulno-lunate joint space visualizes the Ulna (1), the Lunate (2), the TFCC (3), the extensor carpi ulnaris tendon (ECU) is most superficial.

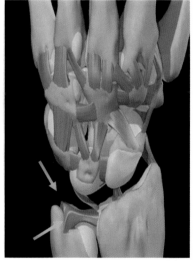

Fig.2 TFCC is an articular dsc, thick at the periphery, and thin centrally.

1. Place the probe in an oblique plane to the long axis of the arm. ***The patient's wrist will be in radial deviation to open the joint space.*** The left boney landmark is the ulna. The cortical outline of the lunate will be to the right of the ulna.

2. The TFC *Complex* is aptly named because it is the aggregate/grouping of six (6) structures. Two of which are the articular disc, and the meniscus homologue. The remaining four (4) are considered part of the ulnocarpal extrinsic ligamentous group. A more dorsal approach, with the wrist in radial deviation (fig 1), will primarily visualize the articular disc ,(fig 2 & 3).

3. The TFCC will be a homogeneous, dense, triangular structure seen within the two boney landmarks. Pathology of fibrocartilage is describeb by anechoic/black lines within the visible articular disc. Fibrocartilage tears are usually irregular or jagged in appearance.

    LABELING : TFCC

THE KNEE

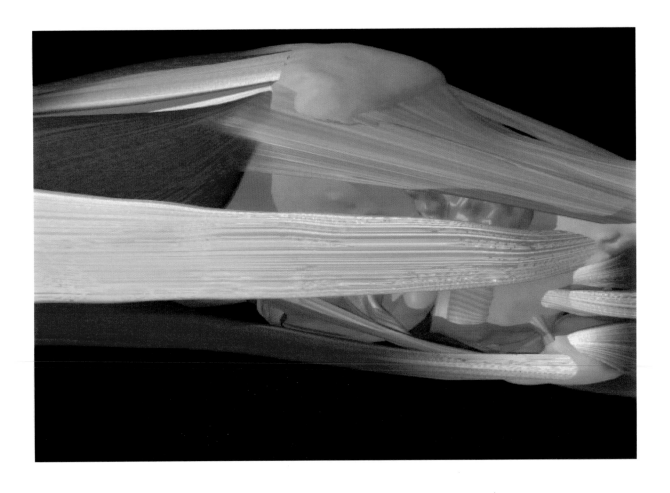

Quadriceps Tendon Longitudinal

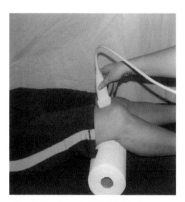

Fig.1 Supine pt. Slight flexion.

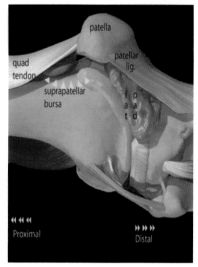

Fig.2 Quad tendon attaches to patella.
Suprapatellar bursa is deep.

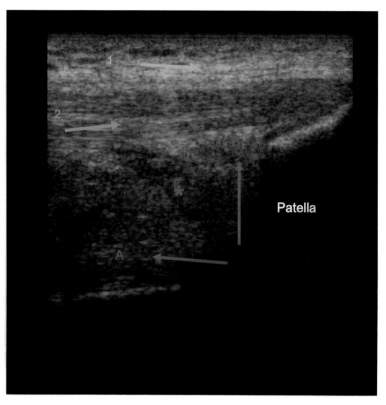

Fig.3 The thick, echogenic tendon is the convergence of four tendons.
(1) Skin, subcutaneous fat, muscle
(2) Quad Tendon
PRE-Femoral Fat Pad (A) and Suprapatellar Fat Pad (B)

1. The patient is supine. The probe is in the longitudinal position with the inferior portion in contact with the patella. The cortical outline of the patella is on the right of the image.

2. The highly echoic quadriceps tendon is composed of three superimposed layers (rectus femoris, vastus lateralis/ medialis ,and vastus intermedius). The suprapatellar bursa is an anechoic fissure that divides the pre-femoral fat pad from the suprapatellar fat pad.

3. Noting the normal presence of two (2) fat pads (fig 2), will help the examiner evaluate the quadriceps tendon. The suprapatellar bursa is continuous with the joint capsule. Effusion of the bursa is seen as it fills a potential space between the two fat pads. (*)

   LABELING: QUAD LONG

Quadriceps Tendon Transverse

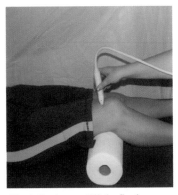

Fig.1 Supine pt. Slight flexion.
Transverse, just proximal to patella.

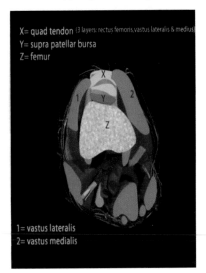

X= quad tendon (3 layers: rectus femoris,vastus lateralis & medius)
Y= supra patellar bursa
Z= femur

1= vastus lateralis
2= vastus medialis

Fig.2 Cross sectional anatomy

1 = RECTUS FEMORIS

2 = VASTUS LATERALIS & MEDIALIS

3 = VASTUS INTERMEDIUS

QUADRICEPS TRANSVERSE

Fig.3 Separation of the three layers can be seen.

1. The patient is in the supine position. The probe is placed in a transverse position just slightly proximal to the patella (on the right knee, left side of monitor is lateral on patient).

2. The cross section of the quadriceps tendon is a large ovoid echogenic area just above the bony shadow of the patella.

3. Separations of the three layers may seen as in the image above. Suprapatellar bursal effusions seen on long axis views, can be tracked to either the medial or lateral aspect.

LABELING: QUAD TRAN

Patellar Tendon Longitudinal

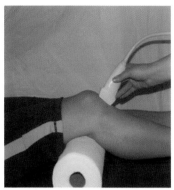

Fig.1 Supine pt. Slight flexion.
Longitudinal distal to patella.

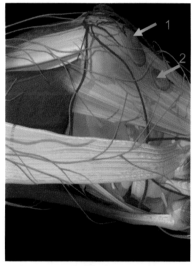

Fig.2 Note the presence of two (2)
Subcutaneous patellar bursae.
PRE– patellar (1)
INFRA-patellar (2)

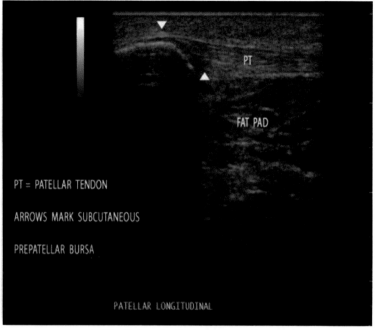

PT = PATELLAR TENDON

ARROWS MARK SUBCUTANEOUS

PREPATELLAR BURSA

PATELLAR LONGITUDINAL

Fig. 3 Longitudinal patellar tendon.
Pre-patellar bursa (between white arrows)
Hint: thicker layer of gel helps "float the probe" , and compress fluid.

1. The patient is supine. Place the probe in the longitudinal position with the proximal portion in contact with the patella. It's boney cortex is seen on the left of the image.

2. The patellar tendon is the thick echogenic structure to the right of the patella. Deep to the patella is the infrapatellar fat pad.   fig. 3
    The subcutaneous prepatellar bursa is situated on top of the lower half of the patella, between the patella and the overlying skin. It is a thin anechoic area between the arrows on the image above.   fig 3

3. NOTE: Fluid in the subcutaneous bursae is easily compressed with probe pressure. It is helpful to use a thicker layer of ultrasound gel over the bursa, and "float the probe".

LABELING: PAT LONG

3 Patellar Bursae

2 Subcutaneous (on top of the tendon)

*Prepatellar= attached to patella
Housemaid 's Knee

*Infrapatellar=Sub-Q, distal, but on top of the tendon
Vicar 's Knee and Jumper 's Knee

1 Deep Infrapatellar (beneath the tendon)
Osgood-Schlatter' s disease
Pathologic due to a traction avulsion injury at the tendon insertion on the tibial tubercle.

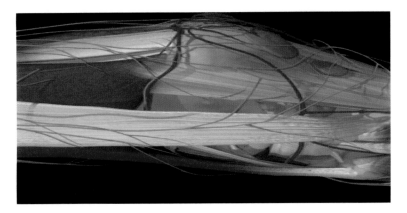

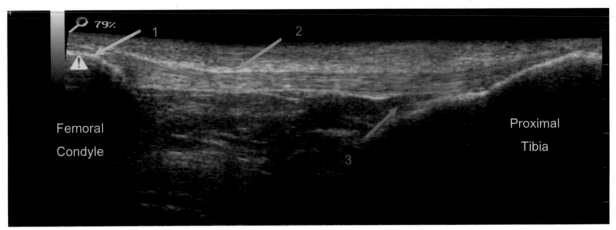

Fig.1 Normal panoramic view of the patellar tendon from origin to insertion
Locations for the 3 patellar bursae. Bursae are "potential spaces" and not visible on this image.
Pre-patellar (1), Infra-patellar (2), DEEP Infra-patellar (3)

Patellar Tendon Transverse

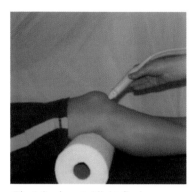

Fig.1 Supine pt. Slight flexion.
Transverse distal to patella

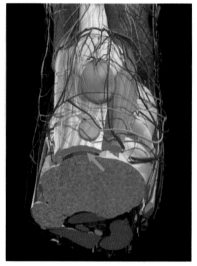

Fig.2 the two subcutaneous bursa
are evident. Note the more distal
Deep Infrapatellar bursa (arrow)

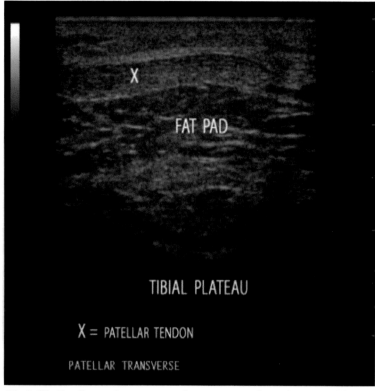

X

FAT PAD

TIBIAL PLATEAU

X = PATELLAR TENDON

PATELLAR TRANSVERSE

Fig.3 The Patellar tendon presents a homogenous, echogenic pattern (X),
with the marbled appearance of the Infrapatellar fat pad deep to it.

1. The patient is in supine position. The probe is placed in the transverse orientation just slightly below the patella.

2. The tendon is seen in cross section just below the skin. The marbled structure deep the tendon is the infrapatellar fat pad. The subcutaneous prepatellar bursa is not usually seen on this image unless there is distention due to fluid. See previous page referring to bursa.

3. The boney landmark of the tibial plateau ,and the anechoic hyaline cartilage are easily visualized.

LABELING: PAT TRANS

Lateral Collateral Ligament Longitudinal

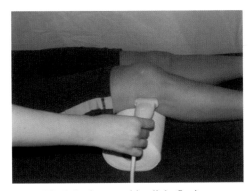

Fig.1 Supine pt. with slight flexion.
Probe is BELOW the IT band

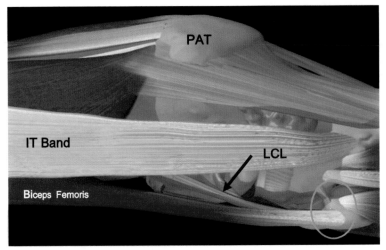

Fig.2 The biceps femoris overlies the LCL.
Both the BF and LCL attach on the fibular head. (hi-lited area)

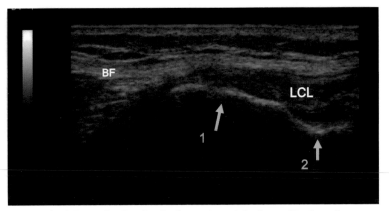

Fig. 3 Boney landmarks: 1= femoral condyle, 2= popliteal notch
The LCL is **hypo**-echoic to the overlying **hyper**-echoic, fibrillar BF tendon

1. The patient is in the supine position. Some internal rotation of the knee maybe necessary.

2. To be certain the LCL is being visualized, place the probe longitudinally on the lateral knee, <u>below</u> the IT Band. Using the boney landmarks of the femoral condyle and the popliteal notch will allow precise positioning to see the LCL. Fig 3

3. The LCL is deep to the brighter, more echogenic biceps femoris tendon. Fig 3

4. After the ligament is identified, it can be traced to the fibular attachment. This is the area most LCL pathology is occurs, most commonly due to excessive varus stress to the knee. A torn LCL will allow the biceps femoris to sag into the void created by the tear.

LABELING: LCL LONG

Lateral Collateral Ligament Transverse

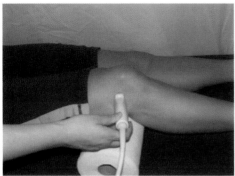

Fig 1 Supine pt. with slight flexion.

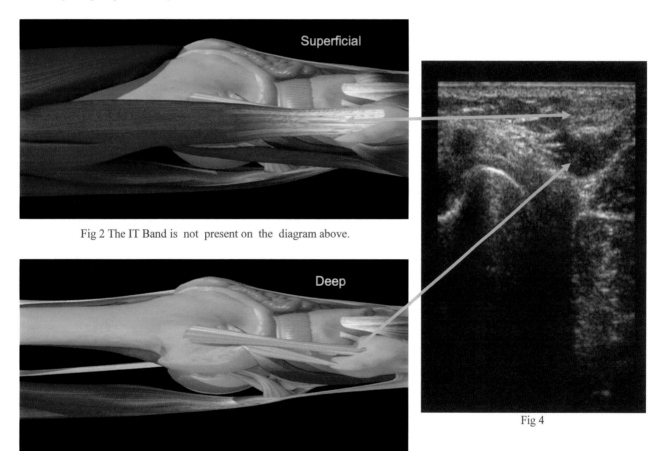

Superficial

Fig 2 The IT Band is not present on the diagram above.

Deep

Fig 4

Fig 3 The LCL is seen with the Biceps Femoris removed

1. The patient is in the supine position. Some internal rotation of the knee maybe necessary. Turn the probe into the short axis of the leg.

2. The biceps femoris tendon and LCL are seen in cross-section. Fig 4

LABELING: LCL TRANS

Medial Collateral Ligament Longitudinal

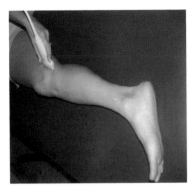

Fig 1 Supine pt. with external rotation

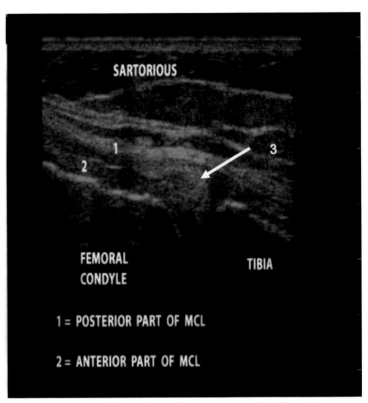

SARTORIOUS

FEMORAL CONDYLE   TIBIA

1 = POSTERIOR PART OF MCL

2 = ANTERIOR PART OF MCL

Fig 3 Anterior and posterior portions are seen proximally on image.
Peripheral margin of medial meniscus is hyper-echoic triangle (3)

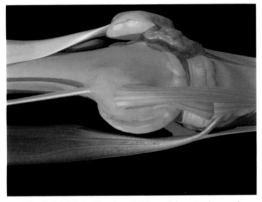

Fig 2 MCL is flat, band-like with anterior and posterior portions, giving a tri-laminar appearance

1. The patient is in the supine position with the knee externally rotated, exposing the medial aspect of the knee. Place the probe in the longitudinal orientation, with the mid-portion at the joint space between the boney landmarks of the femoral condyle and the tibia.

2. The MCL is a strong, flat, band-like ligament consisting of two parts:an anterior band and a posterior band. Overlying the medial collateral ligament will be the musculotendinous portion of the sartorius.

3. The two parts are not physically separate. Two hyperechoic bands are separated by a darker/ hypoechoic area. Sometimes a bursa lies deep to the anterior part separating it from the underlying joint capsule and meniscus. (No bursa is seen on image above)

4. The distal attachment of the MCL is 5-7 cm below the joint. It is at this level a Pes Anserinus bursa may be visible. The Pes Anserinus tendon is a conjoined tendon of the semitendinosus, gracilis, and sartorious tendons. It will be superficial to the MCL at it's distal portion. An extended field of view image is on the following page.

   LABELING : MCL LONG

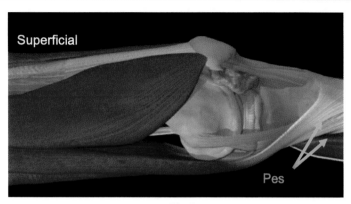

Fig 1

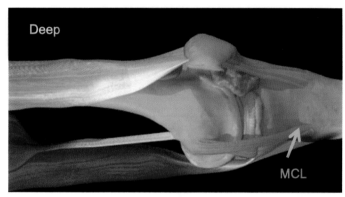

Fig 2

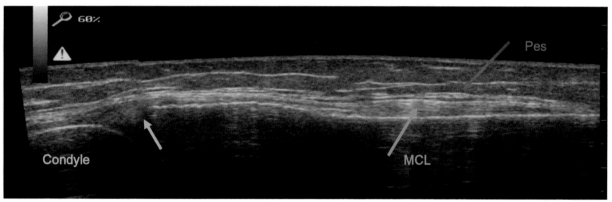

Fig 3

The Pes Anserinus tendon (fig 1) is a conjoined tendon comprised of the **semitendinosus, gracilis, and sartorious** tendons. It will be superficial to the MCL (fig 2) at it's distal portion.

On the image above (fig 3), the thicker MCL is seen directly on top of the tibial cortex. An almost imperceptible anechoic/black line is noted between the MCL, and the very thin pes anserine tendon. This anechoic fissure is the pes anserine bursa.

Lateral Meniscus Longitudinal
Postero-lateral Approach

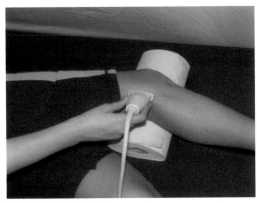

Fig 1 Lateral decubitus pt. with varus stress applied to extended knee.

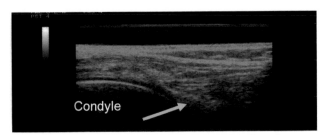

Fig 3a Uniformly hyperechoic triangle of the lateral meniscus is seen between the femoral condyle and the tibia

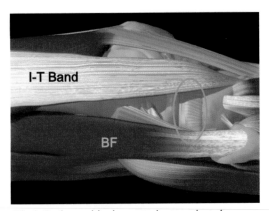

Fig 2 Probe positioning anterior to or just above the fibular head, visualizes LM (hi-lited).

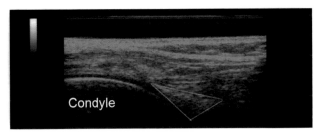

Fig 3b Peripheral margin of lateral meniscus outlined

1. For lateral meniscus scanning a pillow under the patient's knee provides varus stress to open the joint space for optimum viewing of the meniscus.

2. Place the probe on the postero-lateral aspect of the knee in a slightly oblique, longitudnal plane.

3. Aim the probe in a postero-anterior direction. There is an interval between the biceps femoris tendon and the iliotibial tract (see diagram above) which allows visualization of the peripheral margin of the lateral meniscus.

4. The meniscus is a uniformly hyperechoic triangle between the femoral condyle and the tibial bone shadows. Anechoic, irregular lines seen within the visible meniscus are sonographic criteria for meniscal tears.

LABELING: LM LONG

Medial Meniscus Longitudinal
Postero-medial Approach

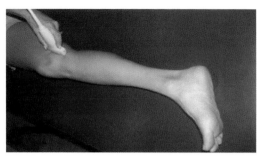

Fig 1 Supine pt. with
external rotation

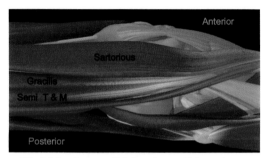

Fig 2 Muscle superficial to the medial meniscus

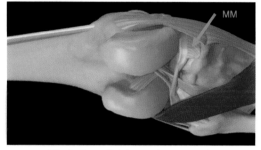

Fig 3 Superficial muscle removed .

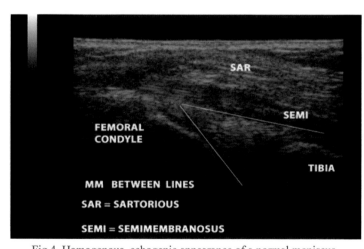

Fig 4 Homogenous, echogenic appearance of a normal meniscus.

1. The patient is supine, and externally rotating the leg for the medial meniscus examination.

2. Place the probe on the postero-medial aspect of the knee in a longitudinal and slightly oblique plane. Aim the sound beam in a postero-anterior direction.

3. The medial meniscus is made of C-shaped cartilage like the lateral meniscus. Look for the uniformly echogenic triangular presence of the meniscus between the femur and the tibia.

4. Muscles overlying the meniscus:
    Superficially: Sartorius
Deep to Sartorius: Semimembranosus

LABELING: MM LONG

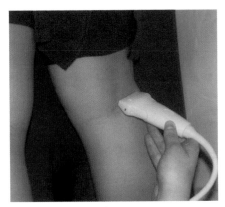

Fig 1 Prone pt.
Small pillow/bolus under the foot suggested

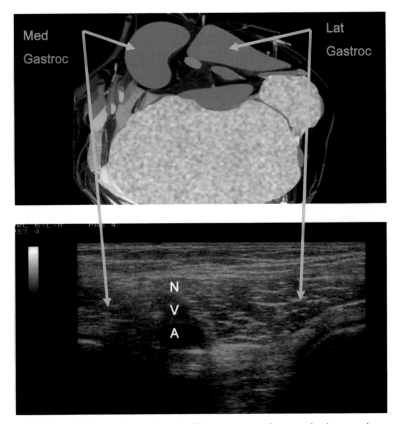

Med Gastroc

Lat Gastroc

N
V
A

Fig 2 The medial and lateral heads of the gastrocnemius muscles in x-section.
N= Tibial Nerve, V= Popliteal Vein, A= Popliteal Artery

1. The patient is prone for the examination of the popliteal fossa. A small bolus under the foot can help relax the skin of the posterior knee. Place the probe in the transverse orientation in the center of the fossa. Fig 1

2. Placing the probe in a somewhat "proximal" portion of the popliteal fossa, the lateral and medial femoral condyles will be the boney landmarks. The heads of the medial and lateral gastrocnemius muscles are viewed in cross-section. Fig 2

3. A true Baker's cyst arises in the margin between the medial gastroc and the semi-membranosus. They are typically not found subcutaneously, but deeper in the inter-muscular margin. A baker's cyst will present with a tell-tale "neck", which is it's origin.

4. Figure 2 also visualizes the <u>pulsatile</u> popliteal artery and the <u>compressible</u> vein, along with the more superficial <u>ovoid</u> (and somewhat medially located) tibial nerve.

LABELING: POP FOSSA TRANS (popliteal fossa transverse)

THE ANKLE and FOOT

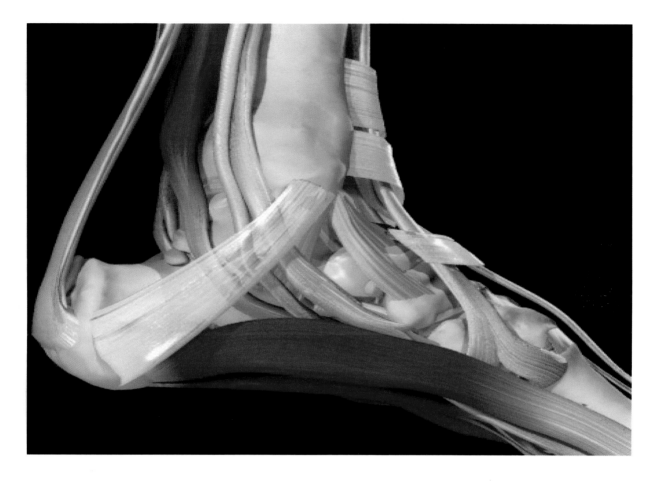

The foot has become one of the most important areas for musculoskeletal ultrasound, rivaling the shoulder for frequency of referral. "

" Many patients present with symptoms localized to particular areas of the foot ,and in these instances ultrasound plays an important role in differential diagnosis. "

Eugene G. McNally, FRCR,FRCPI
Consultant Musculoskeletal Radiologist
Nuffield Othopaedic Centre and John Radciffe Hospitals
Oxford, UK

Ankle: Anterior Longitudinal
Medial of true midline

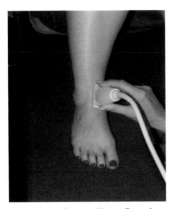

Fig 1 Supine pt. Knee flexed.
No dorsi/plantar flexion
Slightly medial of midline.

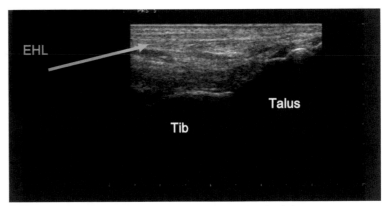

Fig 3 The medial portion of the tibio-talar joint.
No extensor retinaculum should seen.

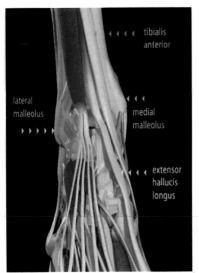

Fig 2 EHL and TA are adjacent
Localize EHL by extension of 1st digit

1. The patient should be supine, with the knee flexed, and the foot flat on the exam table. No dorsi flexion or plantar flexion. The probe is in long axis, medial of midline, and anterior to the medial malleolus. The tibio-talar joint is visualized.

2. The extensor hallucis longus and the tibialis anterior tendons are closely approximated. The tibialis anterior is medial and slightly superficial to the extensor hallucis. To distinguish between them, manually extend the first digit, and watch for the sliding movement of the extensor tendon.

3. Pathology and injury of these tendons is not common. Evaluating the continuity of the tendon fibers, presence of fluid in the tendon sheath, and joint capsule should be noted.

LABELING: EHL / TA LONG

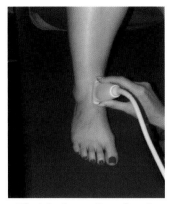

Fig 1 Supine pt. Knee flexed.
No dorsi/plantar flexion
At true midline.

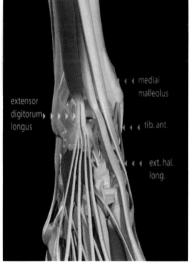

Fig 2 The thickest portion of the EDL
lies deep to the extensor retinaculum.
(Retinculum not on this diagram)

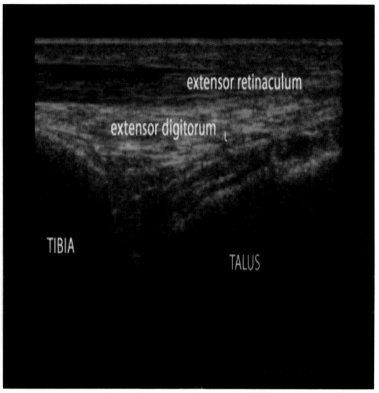

Fig 3 Tibio-talar joint is visualized.
Superficial extensor retinaculum is hypoechoic.
EDL is deeper and hyperechoic

1. The patient should be supine, with the knee flexed, and the foot flat on the exam table. No dorsi flexion or plantar flexion. The probe is in long axis, at the midline. The tibio-talar joint is visualized. Fig 1

2. The extensor digitorum longus muscle becomes tendon, and passes over the anterior ankle joint lateral to the extensor hallucis longus, EHL. Fig 2

3. The extensor digitorum longus tendon is deep to the extensor retinaculum. The tendon is more echogenic/brighter than the retinaculum. Fig 3

LABELING: EDL LONG

Ankle: Anterior Transverse

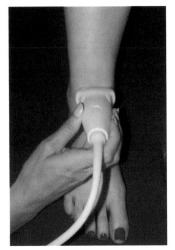

Fig 1 Supine pt. Knee flexed.
No dorsi/plantar flexion
Short axis probe

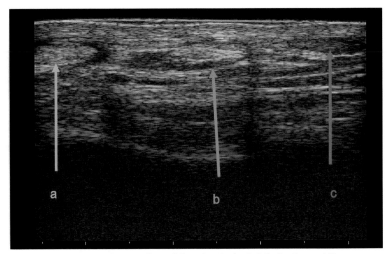

Fig 3 The cortical outline of the talus is the bright horizontal line.
The EDL (a), EHL (b), TA (c) are 3 ovoid structures .
Joint effusion is indicated by a 3mm or larger joint space.

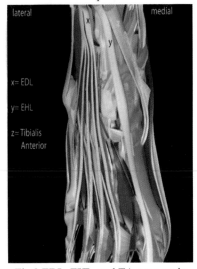

Fig 2 EDL, EHL, and TA are seen in
cross-section as they pass over the
tibio-talar joint

Anterior Ankle Observations

1) Joint effusion, synovitis. Greater than 3mm joint space measurement.

2) Cortical integrity of tibia and talus.

3) Anechoic hyaline cartilage thickness.

4) Extensor tendons intact ? Edematous ?

1. The patient should be supine, with the knee flexed, and the foot flat on the exam table. No dorsi flexion or plantar flexion. The probe is in short axis. The tibio-talar joint is visualized. Fig 1

2. Reading from lateral to medial, the three (3) ovoid structures are the EDL, EHL, and TA. Fig 3

3. The anechoic line of hyaline cartilage identifies the tibio-talar joint space. A measurement of greater than 3mm is sonographic criteria for anterior joint effusion.

LABELING: ANT ANKLE TRANS

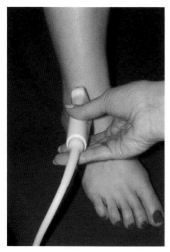

Fig 1 Supine pt. Knee flexed.
Long axis, slightly oblique

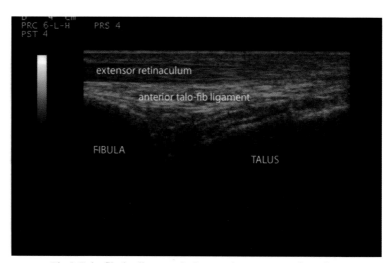

Fig 3 Talo-fibular ligament is deep to the extensor retinaculum.
The fibular malleolus is prominent landmark
TFL is weakest ligament in the ankle

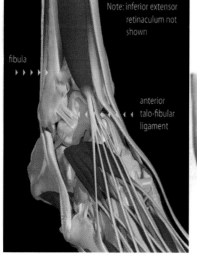
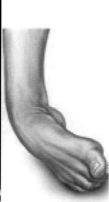

Fig 2 The inferior extensor
retinaculum is not on diagram, but
seen on image at right.

1. The patient should be supine, with the knee flexed, and the foot flat on the exam table. No dorsi flexion or plantar flexion. The probe is in long axis, with a slight lateral-to-medial obliquity to be parallel with the ligament fibers. The talo-fibular joint is visualized, with the fibular malleolus as the prominent boney landmark. Fig 1

2. The talo-fibular ligament is deep to the extensor retinaculum. Figs 1& 2 .It interdigitates with the deeper, anterior joint capsule, and may appear to sag into the joint space .

3. The TFL is the weakest of the ankle collateral ligaments, and most commonly ruptured during inversion injuries Fig 2 offset .

LABELING: TALO-fib LONG

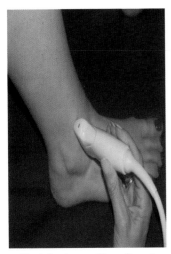

Fig 1 Supine pt. Knee flexed.
Ant/Sup to lateral malleolus
Oblique to see boney landmark

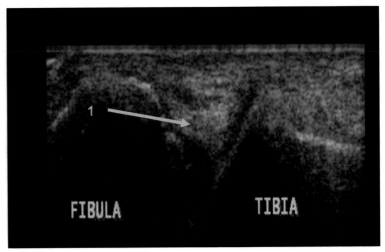

Fig 3 The inter-osseous tibio-fibular ligament (1) is seen between the boney
landmarks of the fibula and tibia. The overlying extensor digitorum longus
muscle is not seen on this image.

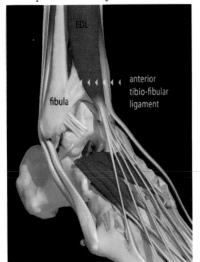

Fig 2 Tib-Fib ligament is
inter-osseous and deep EDL muscle

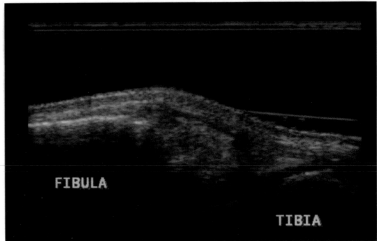

Fig 4 Tibio-fibular ligament image with acoustic stand-off employed

1. The patient should be supine, with the knee flexed, and the foot flat on the exam table. No
    dorsi flexion or plantar flexion. The probe is anterior/superior to the malleolus, in long axis.
    An oblique position is also needed to visualize the inter-osseous Tib-Fib margin. Fig 1

2. The tibio-fibular ligament is seen in cross-section . With the described probe positioning
    here, the sound beam is perpendicular to the ligament fibers.Figs 2 & 3

3. A small but significant minority of lateral ankle sprains may be of sufficient severity to injure
   the distal tibio-fibular syndesmosis, i.e. the ligaments attaching to the distal parts of the tibia
   and fibula. The distinguishing diagnostic factor from a lateral ankle sprain is external rotation
   added to inversion.

LABELING: TIBIO-fib LONG

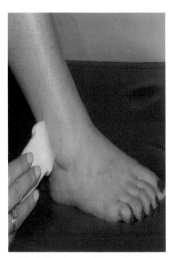

Fig 1 Supine pt. Knee flexed.
Posterior to lateral malleolus
Long Axis

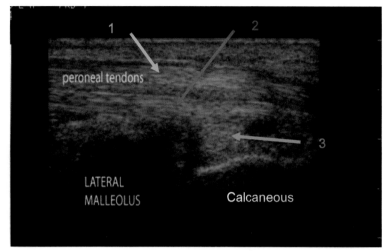

Fig 3 Peroneous longus (1) and brevis (2) , everters of the foot, are easily seen, with brevis deep to longus. The calcaneo-fibular ligament (3) is seen deep to PB.

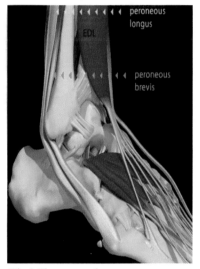

Fig 2 The peroneal compartment tendons run together. Peroneous Brevis is deep to Longus.

1) The foot is flat on the exam table. No extension or eversion of the foot.
   The probe is placed in a longitudinal position, directly behind the lateral malleolus, in line with the lower leg.

2) The peroneal tendons are large tendons of the lateral compartment of the leg. Peroneous longus is superficial, and peroneous brevis is deep. The calcaneo-fibular ligament is seen as an echogenic, rounded structure deep to PB.

3) The peroneal tendons evert the foot (turn it outward), and help plantar flex. Recurrent inversion injuries can produce retinaculum laxity, chronic subluxation, and splitting of PB, easily seen on US.   LABELING: PER LONG

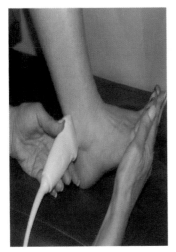

Fig 1 Stress the PL and PB with dorsi-flexion and eversion

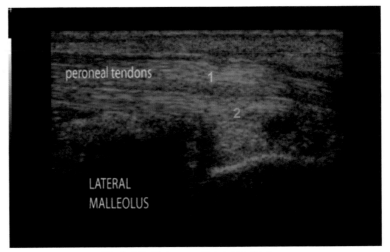

Fig 2 PL (1) is superficial. PB (2) deep.

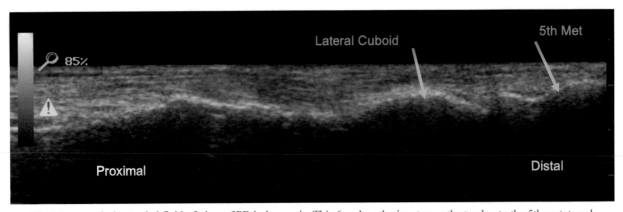

Fig 3 Panoramic / extended field of view of PB in long axis. This 6cm length view traces the tendon to the 5th metatarsal attachment. Splitting of the PB can be a sequelae to repetitive inversion ankle injuries.

1) Applying mild eversion stress may visualize interstitial tears the peroneal tendons.

2) Evaluate the image for tendon subluxation, tears, edema. Breaks or interruption of the boney cortex, especially of the lateral cuboid, 5th metatarsal, can be indicative of stress fractures. Stress fractures can be seen in "twisting type" athletic injuries,but they are more clinically significant in diabetic patients, i.e. Charcot's Neuropathy.

3) Muscle weakness lends itself to tendon rupture, primarily the more superficial PL.

Tarsal Tunnel: Posterior Medial Mallelolus Transverse
Tibialis Posterior, Flexor Digitorum, Tibial Nerve, Flexor Hallucis

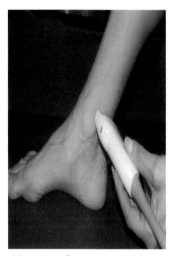

Fig 1 Foot flat on exam table or
with extended knee and
external rotation exposing MM

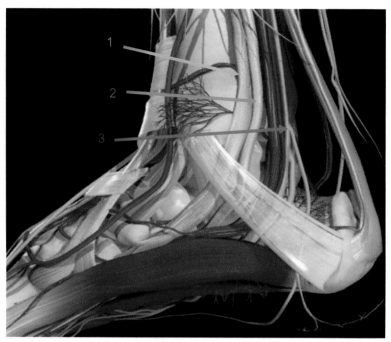

Fig 2 Reading A to P : Tibialis posterior (1), flexor digitorum (2),
Tibial nerve (3). Flexor hallucis is deep to vascular bundle, and not seen

1) The foot can be flat on the exam
exam table, or with extension of
the knee with external rotation, the
medial malleolus is exposed. Probe
is in short axis. The malleolus is the
boney landmark.

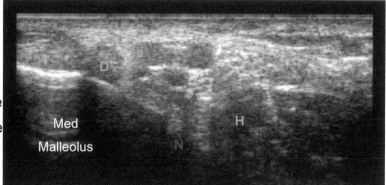

Fig 3 T = tib posterior, D = flexor digitorum, N = tib nerve
H = Flexor hallucis (hypoechoic due to anisotropy)
Acronyms: Tom, Dick, and Nervous Harry
"Mickey Mouse" sign of vascular bundle

2. Two echogenic, ovoid tendons next
to the malleolus are the tibilais
posterior and flexor digitorum.

3) Adjacent to the FDL is the vascular bundle of two veins and one artery. The tibial nerve is the
moderately echoic , round structure next to the (non-compressible with probe pressure) tibial artery.

4) Most pathology in the tarsal tunnel involves the tibialis posterior tendon. Tibial nerve entrapment will present an increased cross-sectional area, best confirmed with comparative imaging.
LABELING: POST MM TRANS

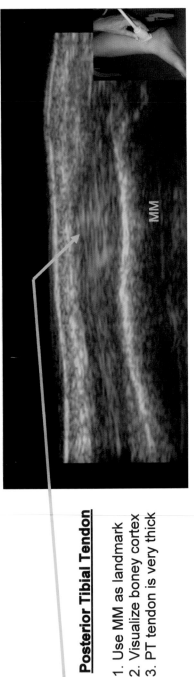

Posterior Tibial Tendon

1. Use MM as landmark
2. Visualize boney cortex
3. PT tendon is very thick

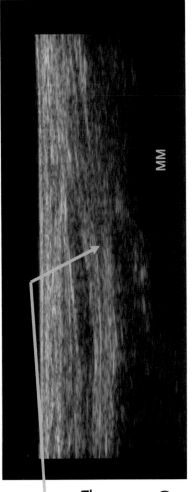

Flexor Digitorum Tendon

1. <u>Aim</u> probe posteriorly
2. FDL is deep to PT
3. Use dynamic maneuver (manually flex 2nd-5th toes)

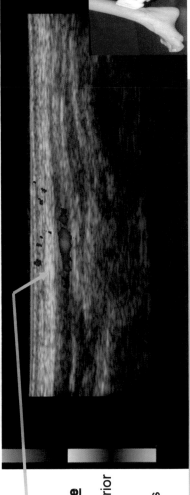

Posterior Tibial Nerve

1. Move probe post-superior
2. Trace pulsatile artery
3. Nerve is superficial to artery. Color flow helps identify artery.

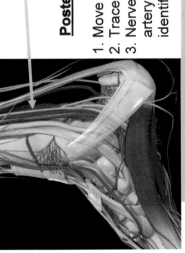

Tarsal Tunnel: Posterior Medial Mallelolus Longitudinal
Tibialis Posterior ,Flexor Digitorum, Tibial Nerve ,Flexor Hallucis

Flexor Hallucis Longitudinal

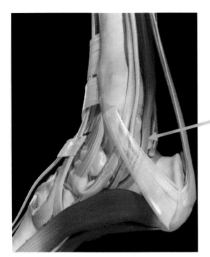

Fig 1 Flexor Hallucis is deep and posterior to vascular-nerve bundle.

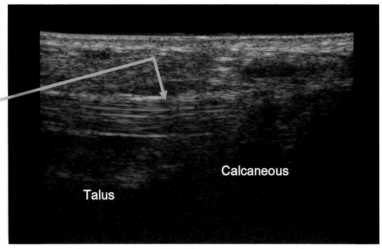

Fig 3 Moving the long axis oriented probe posterior-ward from the MM reveals the talus and calcaneous as boney landmarks. Flexor hallucis is a thick, echogenic tendon. Manual flex of 1st toe helps confirm.

Talus

Calcaneous

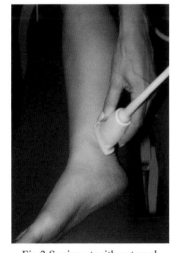

Fig 2 Supine pt with external rotation. Long axis probe posterior to tibial artery

1) The patient is supine on the exam table, with the knee extended,and the foot externally rotated. The probe is in long axis, and moved posteriorly from the tibial artery, to visualize the talus and calcaneous as the boney landmarks. Fig 1

2) The flexor hallucis longus is a large, thick/broad tendon. Care should be taken to visualize the tendon, and not the muscle due to an incorrect superior/proximal probe position. Fig 2 & 3

3) A variety of pathologies affect the FHL. Posterior impingement syndrome. Tenosynovitis at the talus groove. Pseudocyst formation causing triggering of the toe. Longitudinal tears. Pathology is common in dancers and activities creating torsional stress to the hallux.

LABELING: FHL LONG

Achilles Tendon Longitudinal
@ the Insertion

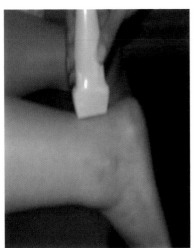

Fig 1 Prone or kneeling pt.
Long axis probe placement

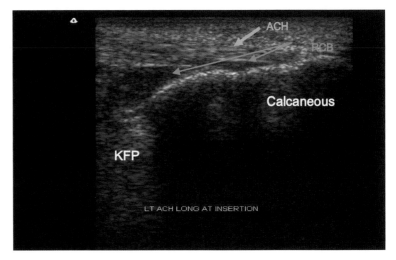

Fig 3 Long axis view of Achilles tendon(ACH) at insertion. Retrocalcaneal bursa (RCB) ,anterior/deep, to tendon is inflamed. Kager's fat pad (KFP) is mixed echoes deep to bursa, which adds support and protection to the tendon

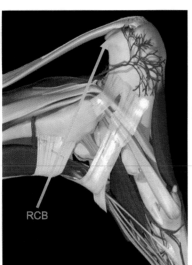

Fig 2 Note the "antierior" position of the retrocalcaneal bursa (RCB) to the ACH. Hindfoot pain may be bursa and/or tendon. Ultrasound imaging allows distinction to be made.

1) The patient is prone or kneeling into a chair, and the probe placed in long axis at the tendon insertion. The calcaneous is the boney landmark. Fig 1

2) The Achilles is large and easily identified by it's dense fibrillar pattern Fig 3. The anechoic area adjacent to the calcaneal cortex is the Retro-calcaneal bursa. A subcutaneous adventitial bursa, on the superficial margin of the Achilles is a frequent observation. It may become inflamed from calcaneal pressure or heel counter irritation. (heel counters are shoe inserts designed to reinforce the heel cup) Kager's fat pad occupies the triangle by the same name. Fibrous connections to the tendon provide proximal stabilization for the Achilles.

Injuries to the Achilles tendon are extremely common in weightbearing sports. Although the term ' t endonitis ' is often used, the most common histopathological finding is that of degeneration within the tendon substance, with no evidence of inflammation. Partial tears and complete rupture of the tendon usually occur on the background of underlying degeneration. However, inflammation does occur in the paratenon. The term tendinopathy should therefore be used to cover the range of pathologies that affect the Achilles. Peritendinitis should be used to describe the inflammatory changes that occur in the paratenon while tendinosis should refer to the degenerative disease of the tendon.Tendinosis is often asymptomatic and may reflect age-related change and response to years of weightbearing exercise.

LABELING : ACH LONG insert

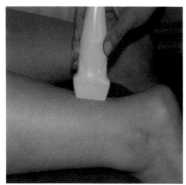

Fig 1 Prone or kneeling pt. Move probe proximally from insertion

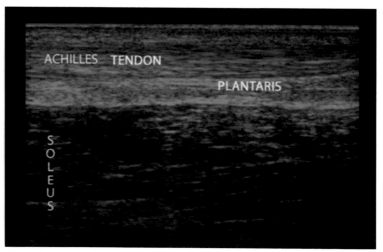

Fig 3 Long axis view of the ACH proximal from insertion. The ACH is superficial. The Plantaris is deep and slightly medial. The darker Soleus muscle is deep to the tendon(s)

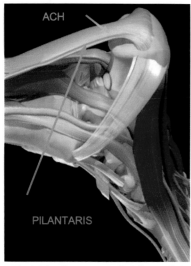

Fig 2 The deeper and slightly medial tendon of Plantaris can be seen. It is much thinner than ACH

Image Tips

* A thickened (> 12-15 mm), fusiform tendon, calcification, and loss of the normal pre-Achilles fat (Kager 's triangle) due to retrocalcaneal bursitis are sonographic criteria for pathology.

* Most ACH tears occur 6-7 CM proximal from insertion

* Ultrasound can demonstrate tendinosis and partial and complete tendon tears with an accuracy.

1) The patient is prone or kneeling into a chair, and the probe is inlong axis, but moved proximally up the leg. The calcaneous is not visible on this image.

2) Position the probe to visualize tendon and muscle.
   a. Achilles tendon will be the most superficial structure
   b. Immediately below the Achilles tendon is the tendon of the plantaris.
   c. Deep to the plantaris will be the soleus muscle.

   NOTE: the muscles of Flexor hallucis longus and flexor digitorum longus are deep to the soleus, but rarely visualized when using high-frequency probes.
   The plantaris tendon is rarely clinically significant. Typically used for tendon grafts.

   LABELING: ACH LONG

Achilles Tendon Transverse

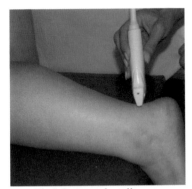

Fig 1 Prone or kneeling pt.
Short axis probe near insertion

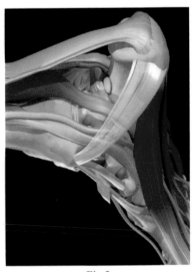

Fig 2

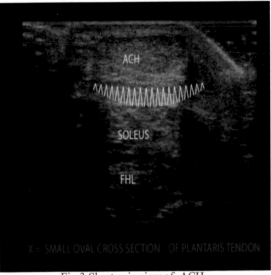

Fig 3 Short axis view of ACH.
Normal appearance is ovoid ,or a concavity on
calcaneal margin producing a reniform or kidney bean
shape.

1) The patient is prone or kneeling into a chair, and the probe is in short axis, near the insertion.

2) Position the probe to visualize tendon and muscle. The echogenic, bristle-like appearance of the Achilles is the most superficial structure. The Plantaris tendon is difficult to visualize in this orientation, but may seen on the medial aspect of the ACH. Mixed echoes typical of skeletal muscle deep to the tendon, is the Soleus.

   NOTE: To minimize lateral and medial margin "edge artifacts" it is necessary to tilt the probe to each side of the tendon to fully examine edges of the tendon.

3) In short axis the Achilles should be ovoid ,or more likely, reniform/ kidney shaped, with the concavity on the calcaneal margin as the tendon rests on the bone.

4) Normal <u>cross-sectional</u> (A to P) measurement for the ACH is 5.5 to 6.5 mm.
   Normal <u>coronal measurement </u> is 9.0 to 13 mm. ⟵⟶
      LABELING : ACH TRANS

Plantar Fascia Longitudinal

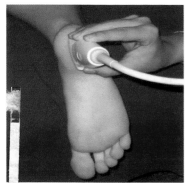

Fig 1 Prone or kneeling pt.
Long axis probe aimed medially

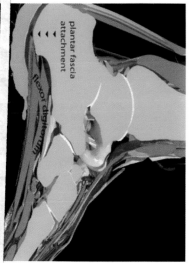

Fig 2 PF attachment in green.
Fat pad superficial
Flexor digitorum deep to PF

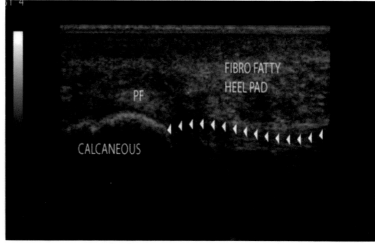

Fig 3 Long axis view of Plantar Fascia
There should NOT be a bursa. Fluid accumulation is abnormal.
> 4mm thickness is criteria for fasciitis.

Image Tips : Risk Factors to PF Injury

1. A sudden increase in sporting activity.

2. A change of running surface.

3. Inadequate arch support and/or cushioning in shoes

4. Tightness of the Achilles tendon.

1)   The patient is prone or kneeling into a chair. The probe is in long axis orientation, angled
medially toward the attachment onto the medial tubercle of the calcaneous. Fig 1

2) Reading the image from the cortical outline to the surface:
a. Plantar Fascia
b. Fibro Fat Pad
Musculature seen deep to the fascia, and distal from the calcaneous, is the flexor digitorum
brevis and abductor minimi. Fig 2 & 3

3.) Plantar fasciitis is an extremely common foot complaint in both the sporting and non-athletic
population. Inflammation of the plantar fascia and the intrinsic muscular attachments of the
hindfoot often manifests itself as localized pain, often exquisite in intensity, at their attachments
onto the medial calcaneal tuberosity.

LABELING : PF LONG

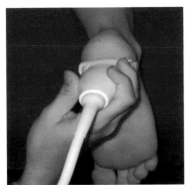

Fig 1 Prone or kneeling pt.
Short axis probe position .
Slight medial "tilt"

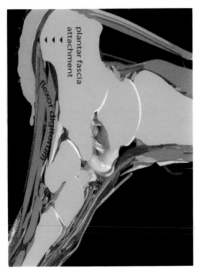

plantar fascia
attachment

flexor digitorum

Fig 2 PF attachment in green.
Fat pad superficial
Flexor digitorum deep to PF

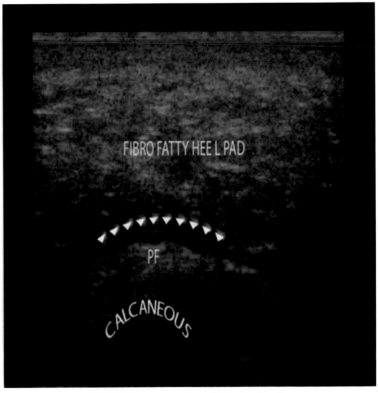

FIBRO FATTY HEE L PAD

PF

CALCANEOUS

Fig 3   Transverse view of Plantar Fascia
Visualize an echogenic arc of the Calcaneous.
Plantar Fascia attachment may be seen on medial tubercle.

1) The patient is prone or kneeling into a chair. The probe is in short axis orientation, tilted
    medially toward the attachment onto the medial tubercle of the calcaneous. Fig 1

2) The plantar fascia is an echogenic,focal point on the medial margin of the calcaneous.

3) Plantar Fascia measurements are performed on longitudinal views, and therefore considered t
    the more valuable diagnostic view.

4) Examination confirms localized tenderness on the medial aspect of the heel around the origin of
    the fascia. The combination of the tender site and early morning stiffness distinguishes plantar
    fasciitis from other causes of inferior heel pain. Ultrasound can be used to guide local
    injection into the fascia.

LABELING : PF TRANS

Distal Plantar Foot
Flexor Hallucis and Plantar Plate Longitudinal

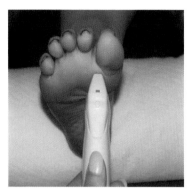

Fig 1 Supine pt with long axis probe position at 1st MPJ .

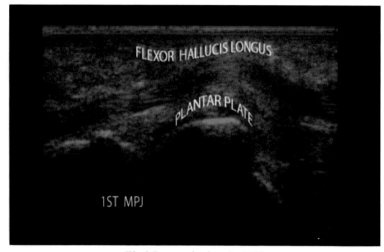

Fig 3 Long axis view 1st MPJ
FHL is most superficial. Plantar Plate (PP) is deep to FHL.
Joint capsule is deep to PP. Scanning in the true midline of the MPJ
is necessary to scan between the medial and lateral sesamoid bones.

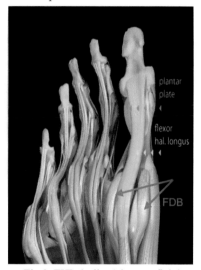

Fig 2 FHL (yellow) is superficial
to PP (green)
flexor digitorum brevis, FDB

Image Tip

Hyperextension injuries to the first toe can avulse

the plantar ligament, tearing some of the metatarsal

head away. Hence the term…

Plantar Plate Fracture

1. Place the probe in a longitudinal position at the 1st MPJ. It is important to scan in the true midline of the 1st MPJ. Slight medial or lateral beam angulation will visualize the medial or lateral sesamoid bones; which are embedded in the Flexor Hallucis Brevis tendons. Fig 1 & 2

2. The flexor hallucis longus is the most superficial structure. Fig 3

3. The plantar plate (i.e. plantar ligament) is a thick echogenic layer deep to the FHL. Fig 3

4. Just below the plantar plate will be the joint capsule, seen as a dark elliptical area.

5. When examining suspected interdigital pain and neuromas, perform similar images as above, and label appropriately (2 through 5 MPJ). Then use the images with corresponding transverse views as seen on the following page.

LABELING : 1ST thru 5TH MPJ LONG

Distal Plantar Foot Transverse
Interdigital Pain and Neuromas

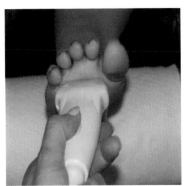

Fig 1 Supine pt with short axis probe at the metatarsal heads.

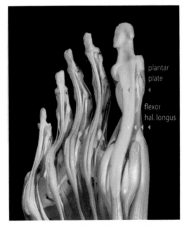

Fig 2 Plantar forefoot showing the plantar plates (yellow) as most superficial structure

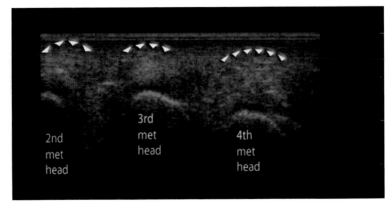

Fig 3 Short axis view of plantar forefoot
Try to visualize three metatarsal heads
NOTE: Homogenous echogenicity of interdigital spaces

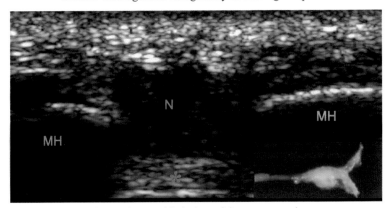

Fig 4 Short axis magnified view of intermetatarsal space.
NOTE: Hypoechoic area, N, BETWEEN the metatarsal heads ,MH

1) Place the probe in short axis across 2-3 metatarsal heads, Fig 3. The cortical outline of the metatarsal heads is the boney landmark. *Make note of homogenous echogenicity within the interdigital spaces,* which is normal due to the accessory collateral ligaments and deep transverse ligaments present in the interosseous margins. Fig 1

2) The plantar ligaments are the most superficial structure to the joint capsule, Fig 2. The deep transverse ligaments, and fan-shaped collateral/suspensory ligaments have fibers that are mostly parallel with the probe, making them readily visible spanning the interdigital spaces, * on Fig 4.

3) Using the transverse and suspensory ligaments as the bottom margin, and the plantar ligaments as the top margin, a hypoechoic oval between the two ligamentous borders is good sonographic criteria for identifying a neuroma. Fig 4

4) **Characteristics of Morton 's Neuroma**: A) 3 rd interspace most common, B) hypoechoic, well-defined, ovoid mass, C) 5-7 mm diameter, D) 80 % middle age females

Upper Extremity Pathology

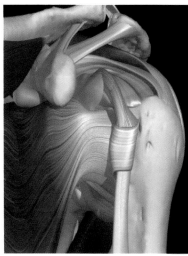

Shoulder

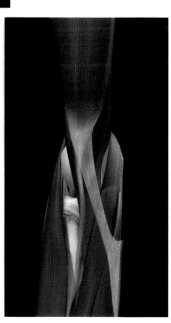

Elbow

Wrist

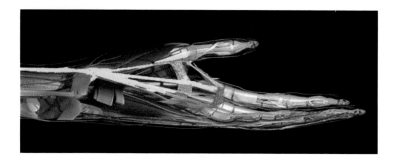

Forward flexion of the arm immediately abuts the SSP against Coraco-Humeral ligament

Resulting in MECHANICAL irritation and ischemia

Prolonged irritation producing tendinopathy & degenerative changes

Fiber Failure which impairs shoulder stability GH joint

Allowing elevation/ superior subluxation of humerus via deltoid contraction

1) Less than 6mm Acromio-humeral separation
in forward flexion position.

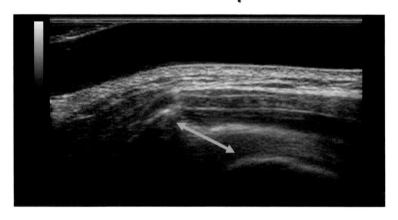

2) Absence of tendon contour & non-visualization

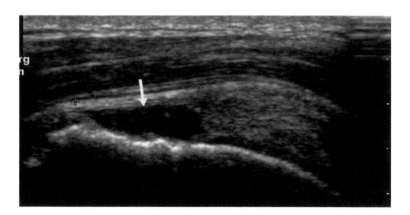

Critical Zone Tear: SSP with retraction

3) Loss of Volume or < 6mm thickness

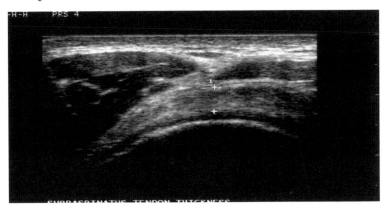

Contralateral measurements suggested

4) Loss of homogenous, echogenic pattern
5) Anechoic areas within the tendon (intrasubstance)

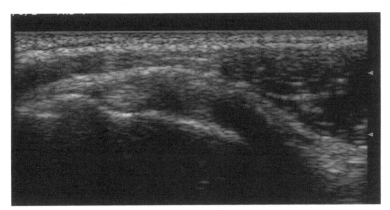

Articular surface SSP tear

6) Loss of contour and non-visualization

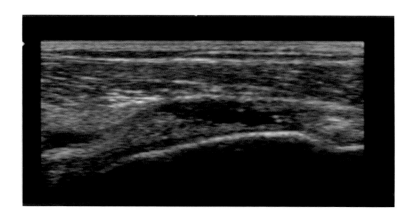

Bursal surface SSP tear

Note for surgeons: A 1 CM tear measured sonographically will present

Larger or wider at arthroscopic surgery due to distention from air and fluid.

The ultrasound measurement is accurate

1) Less than 6mm Acromio-humeral separation in forward flexion position.

2) Absence of tendon contour & non-visualization

3) Loss of Volume or < 6mm thickness

4) Loss of homogenous, echogenic pattern

5) Anechoic areas within the tendon (intrasubstance)

6) Loss of contour and non-visualization

Anatomical images courtesy of Primal Pictures Anatomy Software

**Isolated tears seen in 2 % of cuff tears.
Usually an incidental finding.**

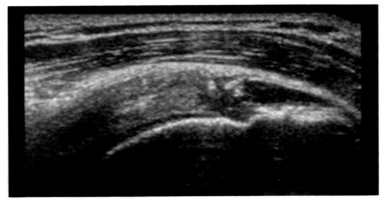

Calcification within the Subscapularis tendon

**Longitudinal view intact SSP tendon
Note the superficial location of the bursa.**

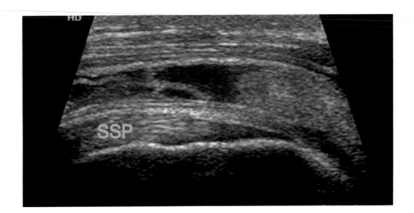

**Hyperechoic foci within the bursa would be indicative of
proliferative or infectious bursitis**

Subcutaneous Lipoma

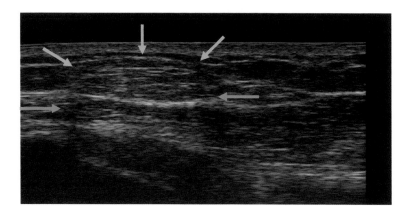

Lipoma sonographically identified in a physician who suspected chronic bursal effusion. Yellow arrows define superficial border. Green arrows identify "edge artifact" of anechoic/black vertical lines, with hyperechoic "posterior enhancement" artifact between.

Active Shoulder Synovitis
Doppler Flow Imaging

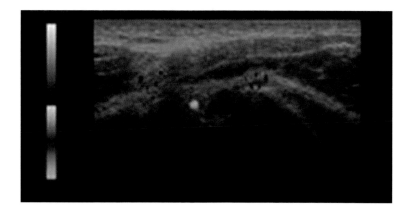

**Transverse of the biceps tendon. Local hyperemia is often associated with focal tendon lesions. Synovial reaction is seen in inflammatory arthropathies. Granulation tissue at sites of healing is vascular.
Doppler imaging presents amplitude of flow as a color signal. Easier to perform than color flow mapping. Not dependent on angle. Fewer artifacts. Detects low amplitude flow.**

Upper Extremity Pathology
Posterior Elbow Effusion

Epitrochlear Effusion

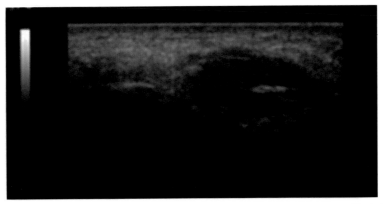

No well-defined joint margin. Large nearly anechoic fluid collection.

Posterior Elbow Capsular Effusion

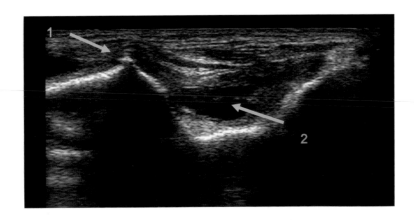

**Transverse image of posterior elbow compartment.
Note the loose cortical fragment at left (1), which is lateral trochlea.
Fluid is intracapsular(2), and the fat pad is displaced superficially.**

Lateral Epicondylitis

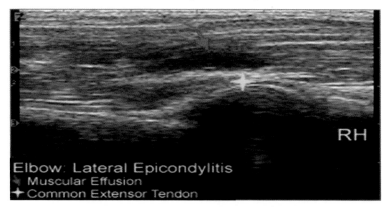

The yellow star visualizes the common extensor tendon as it passes over the radial head. Note the thickness of the common extensor tendon between the green arrows. There is some non-visualization of tendon fibers.

Lateral Epicondylitis

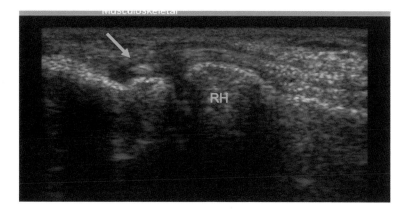

Near full-thickness tear with calcification of Common Extensor. Female. College volleyball player. RH = radial head

Dorsal Ganglion of the Wrist : Transverse

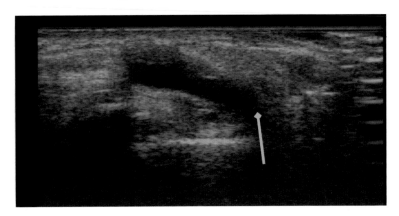

Dorsal ganglia will be located DEEP to the very thin, subcutaneous extensor tendons. May be indicative of carpal instability, as the ganglion is seen emerging from within the carpal bones.
May or may not be painful.

Dorsal Ganglion of the Wrist : Longitudinal

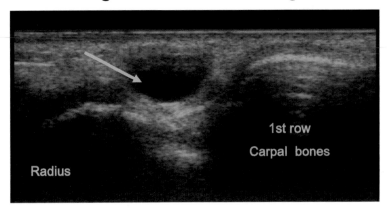

Radius

1st row
Carpal bones

Recurrent dorsal ganglia may demonstrate hyperemia on Doppler Flow. This is not uncommon, and should not be taken as a sign of infection. Doppler not applied to image.

Upper Extremity Pathology
Wrist: Extensor Tenosynovitis

Extensors of the Wrist : Transverse

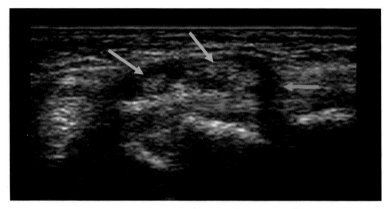

**Note the "Halo sign" indicative of
tenosynovitis. Vertical anechoic lines (green arrow) are
"edge artifact". Note there are two extensors inflamed (yellow arrows).
Common in repetitive stress syndromes**

Extensors of the Wrist : Longitudinal

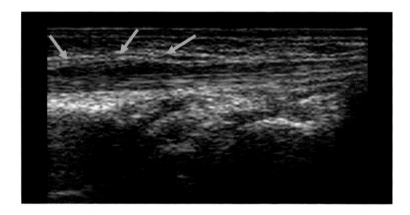

**Fluid in the tendon sheath layers out as
an anechoic sheet on the dorsal aspect of
the tendon. The tendon takes on a fusiform appearance**

Upper Extremity Pathology
TFCC :Triangular Fibrocartilage Complex

TFCC Longitudinal : Abnormal

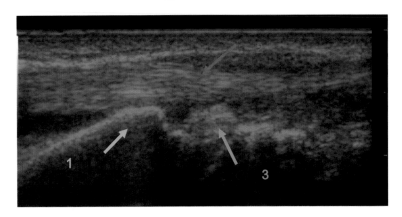

Ulnar Styloid (1)
Extensor Carpi Ulnaris (2)
TFC and radio-ulnar ligament (3)
Loss of contour.
Inconsistent echo-density. Mottled appearance .
Common injury in cases with severe ulnar deviation

TFCC Longitudinal : Normal

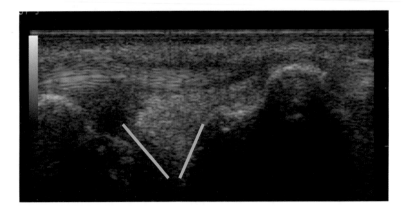

Triangular Shape. Consistent, homogenous echo-density

UCL Longitudinal

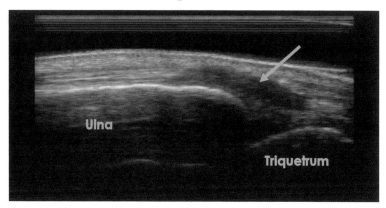

**Left UCL in female ,mid-twenties. Life-long bilateral pain.
Cortex of boney landmarks intact due to no surgical debridement.**

UCL Longitudinal

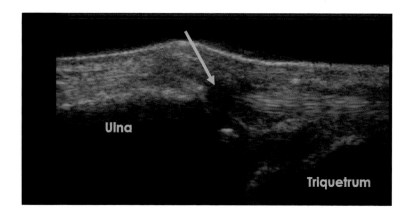

Right UCL ,same patient. 2 years post-debridement.

Note the loss of smooth, intact cortical outline.

There is some non-visualization of ligament due to anisoptropy.

Ligament fiber failure is also present in this chronic case.

Dorsal MCP Longitudinal

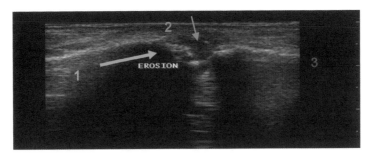

Active rheumatoid arthritis
Cortical eroision (1)
No distinct anechoic cartilage margin (2)
Poorly visible extensor tendon (3)

Synovial Fluid vs Synovial Hypertrophy

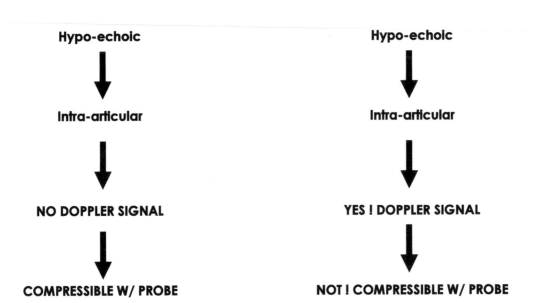

Fluid	Hypertrophy
Hypo-echoic	Hypo-echoic
↓	↓
Intra-articular	Intra-articular
↓	↓
NO DOPPLER SIGNAL	YES ! DOPPLER SIGNAL
↓	↓
COMPRESSIBLE W/ PROBE	NOT ! COMPRESSIBLE W/ PROBE

Lower Extremity Pathology

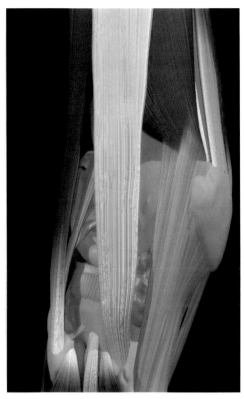

Knee

Foot & Ankle

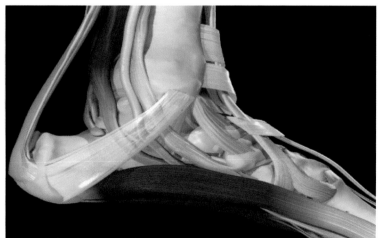

Lower Extremity Pathology
Suprapatellar Bursa Effusion and Quadriceps Rupture

Longitudinal Quadriceps Tendon

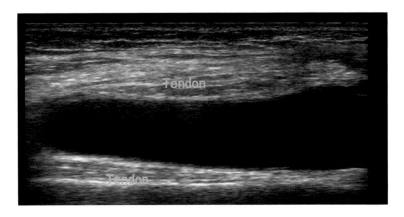

RA patient.
Suprapatellar bursal effusion is dissecting the Quad tendon.
Normal length of the bursa is a mean 22.2 mm
Note the absence of the patella as a landmark on the right side.

Longitudinal Quadriceps Tendon

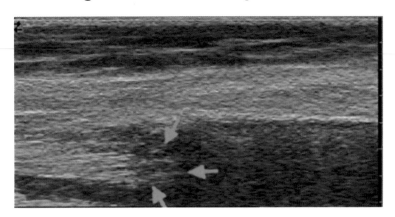

Rupture of deeper portion (vastus lateralis/medialis) of Quad tendon.
This is a disabling injury, often associated with falling while descending stairs or slopes. Extension of the lower leg is not possible.

Longitudinal Patellar Tendon

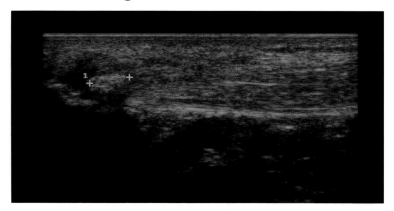

**osteoarthritic male. Two debridements.
Chronic pain.
Note irregular contour of patella, peritendinous fluid, and
small granuloma between cursors.**

Longitudinal LCL

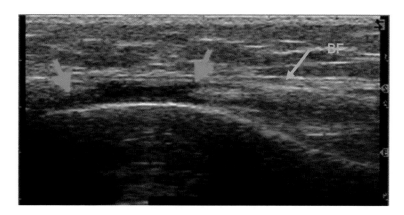

**Note the fibrillar pattern of the hyperechoic, intact Biceps Femoris
Overlying the obvious non-visualization of the deeper LCL**

Longitudinal MCL @ Distal Attachment

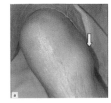

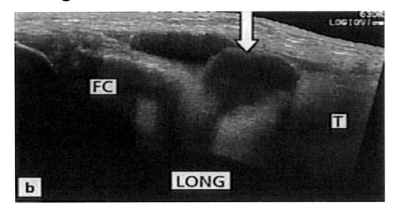

An enlarged, distended bursa
Can be painful and limit knee function.
Ultrasound is able distinguish from a meniscal cyst.
The boney landmark of the femoral condyle, FC and Tibia ,T

Longitudinal MCL @ Distal Portion

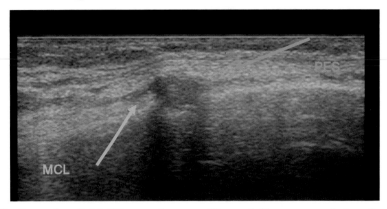

Untreated MCL rupture after skiing accident.
Note irregular proximal end of MCL. Pes Anserinus overlying.
damaged tibial cortex and bone callous formation.

Meniscal Tear Longitudinal

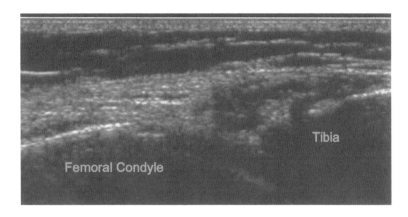

Meniscal tear with complex hypoechoic defects.

Meniscal Cyst Longitudinal

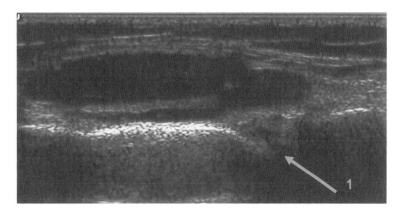

An intra-compartmental cyst adjacent to the meniscus (1) exhibiting a linear, anechoic cleft from a horizontal tear

Lower Extremity Pathology
Baker's Cyst vs Synovial Pouch

Popliteal Fossa Transverse

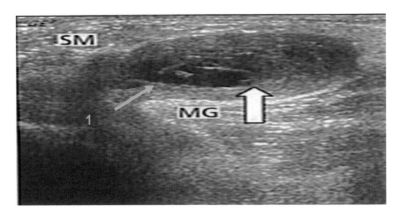

True Baker's cyst ... is INTER-MUSCULAR.
Between the Semimembranosus, and the Medial Gastrocnemius
Originates on the medial side of the Popliteal Fossa
Has a distinct neck (1)

Popliteal Fossa Transverse

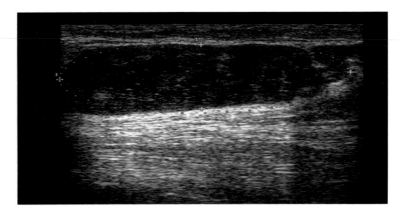

Synovial cysts are subcutaneous and distend the joint capsule.
The fluid –filled cyst is superficial to any visible muscle.

Lower Extremity Pathology
Hamstring Syndrome and Trochanteric Bursitis

Longitudinal at the Gluteal Fold

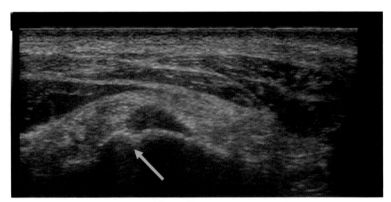

Chronic tendon tautness
**Partial thickness tear and fluid accumulation involving
the Semitendinosis/Biceps Femoris complex in a male
long distance runner. Note cortical depression, suggestive of avulsion.**

Transverse at the Greater Trochanter of the Hip

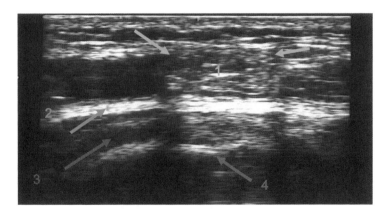

Post-trauma trochanteric bursitis and hematoma
Hematoma and fluid within ITB (1)
Myofascial interface of Gluteus Maximus (2)
Bursal Effusion (3)
Cortex of Greater Trochanter (4)
Note "edge artifact "on both margins of hematoma

Lower Extremity Pathology
Achilles Tendinitis

Transverse Achilles Tendon

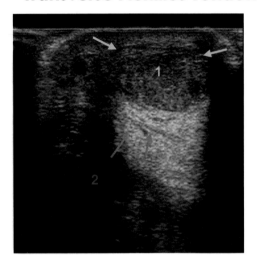

Plump "ball-like" appearance of tendon (1)
(Normal is ovoid or reniform)
Excessive hyperechogenicity of muscle deep to tendon
due to fatty infiltration and mucoid degeneration
Curvilinear lines of muscle tear (2)

Achilles Tendon Longitudinal

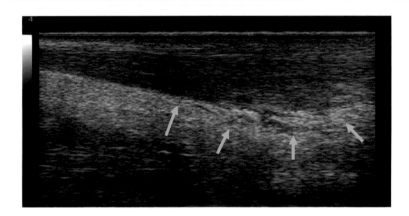

The tendon is hypoechoic and fusiform as it bulges into to the
Weakened portion of the Soleus .

Plantar Fascia Longitudinal

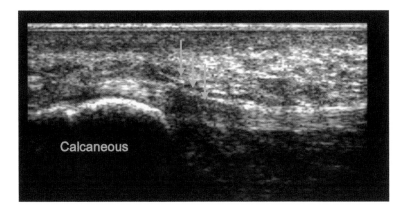

The PF is thickened and hypoechoic near the calcaneal attachment.

1st MPJ Longitudinal

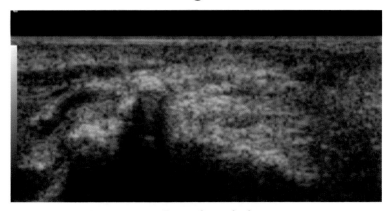

Hyper-extension injury
Plantar ligament is avulsed and displaced toward the skin.
Note posterior shadowing below the ligament .

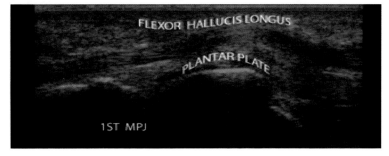

Normal Image

Lower Extremity Pathology
Identifying Neuromas

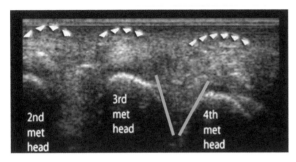

Normal Transverse Plantar Forefoot

Arrows outline the flexor tendons. Note the homogeneous interdigital echoes from the deep transverse and accessory ligaments within the inter-osseous region (yellow lines).

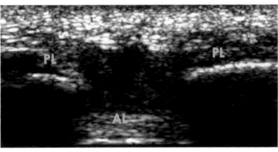

Transverse View: Neuroma

Use the plantar ligaments (PL) as a top or superficial margin (immediately superficial to the joint capsule, and above the cortical outline), and the accessory ligaments (AL) as a bottom margin. A *hypoechoic, ovoid area between the ligament boundaries* is the soft tissue mass or neuroma.

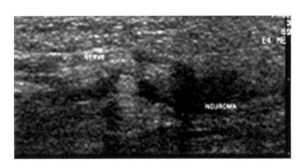

Longitudinal View: Neuroma

Longitudinal view of a neuroma. The hyperechoic nerve can be traced distally to the darker, soft tissue mass. Surgically removed neuroma below.

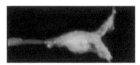

Sample Reports

The following sample reports are presented as examples to aid the doctor and sonographer in developing a complete, yet concise report of findings for musculoskeletal examinations.

The reports are likely to be more extensive than what will be needed on a typical examination, since not every image presented in the extremity protocol is routinely performed on a patient. Please use your own discretion to edit, omit or add to the following sample reports.

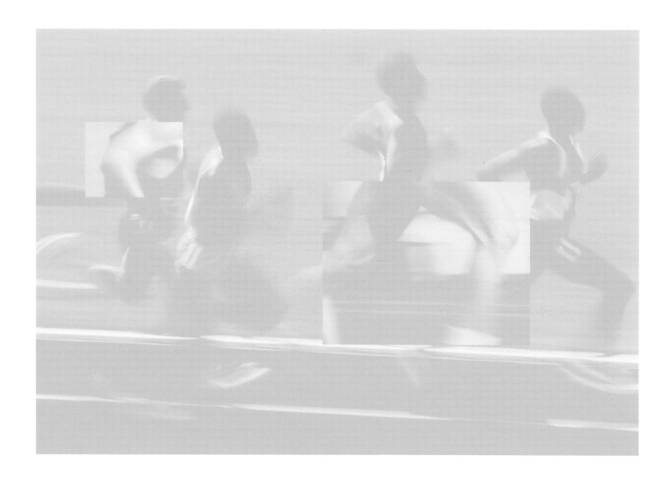

Shoulder

Static real-time views in longitudinal and transverse orientation were obtained on this ___ year old male/female. In transverse view the biceps tendon is hypoechoic and increased in size, measuring ___mm in thickness. (3.0 –3.5 normal). It is well situated in the inter-tubercular groove, no evidence of medial or lateral subluxation. On long axis, the biceps is intact, but remains hypoechoic with a fusiform appearance as it proceeds distally.

On external rotation, the subscapularis tendon appeared intact, not edematous, with no evidence of tenosynovitis nor tendinosis.

The supraspinatus tendon was not thickened (Normal = 4.6-6.0 mm) due to edema, and intact when evaluated in the anterior cuff margin, and at the attachment. The infraspinatus and teres minor tendons were normal. No cortical interruption or irregularity of the humeral head. The humeral hyaline cartilage was ___ mm in thickness below the supraspinatus (Normal = 0.8mm) .

The rotator cuff interval did not demonstrate increased supraspinatus or subscapularis margin effusion. Normal = 3.0 and 3.0 mm

Dynamic imaging to evaluate for impingement demonstrated smooth, unobstructed movement of the supraspinatus beneath the acromion with patient flexion/abduction.

Bilateral acromo-clavicular joint images do not reveal sonographic criteria of ligament laxity or shoulder separation.

Glenoid Labrum and inferior gleno-humeral ligament interruption or tear were not demonstrated.

Sample Reports
Elbow

Static real-time views in longitudinal and transverse orientation were obtained on this ___ year old male/female. There is no sonographic indication of anterior joint capsule effusion or fluid collection. Anterior joint capsule thickness is < 2mm, and the fat pad is not displaced superficially as seen with fluid accumulations. The radial head and trochlear notch cortical outlines are smooth and intact. No visible bone spurs or joint mice.

The biceps tendon is normal on short axis at the cubital fossa. The brachilais muscle, deep to the biceps tendon, demonstrates normal muscle fascia and fibers. No evidence of edema, rupture or hematoma. At it's radial attachment, the tendon is intact, not hypoechoic as seen with inflammation.

Antero-lateral elbow images demonstrate normal cortical outline of the humeral capitellum and radial head. The hyaline cartilage is well visualized. The annular ligament demonstrates homogenous echo signal, and the radial recess does not appear to be distended from effusion. The common extensor tendon is seen intact, attached to the lateral epicondyle, and not inflamed. No visible synovium. Overlying brachio-radialis and extensor carpi radialis muscles are normal.

Medial images demonstrate a normal humero-ulnar outline of the trochlea and trochlear notch. The visible ulnar collateral ligament is homogenous in echogenicity, no apparent tear, rupture or edema. The ulnar nerve is seen in it's normal position, adjacent and posterior to the medial epicondyle. No subluxation on dynamic imaging. Cross sectional area is < 7.5 mm.

Posterior imaging demonstrates normal triceps tendon and muscle. No posterior capsule effusion or bursal fluid accumulation.

Sample Reports
Wrist and Hand

Static real-time views in longitudinal and transverse orientation were obtained on this ___ year old male/female. An acoustic stand-off was/was not utilized.

Palmar images demonstrate normal, intact flexor tendons with no synovitis. On short axis, the median nerve measures __mm. Normal range for a male/female is 7-9 mm. Comparative imaging of the contra-lateral median nerve produced a cross-sectional area of __ . On longitudinal view, the median nerve was/was not hypoechoic, enlarged or fusiform proximal to the flexor retinaculum, and entrance into the carpal tunnel.

Dorsal images demonstrate the extensor tendons in individual compartments with no enlargement due to inflammation. They are intact on long axis. No ganglion cyst is visualized. The dorsal aspect of the 1st metacarpal joint in long axis reveals normal extensor pollicus tendons. Proximal to the extensor retinaculum, the extensor pollicus brevis and abductor pollicus longus are not edematous as seen in De Quervain's tenosynovitis. More distally, and on the ulnar aspect ,at the 1st MPJ, the ulnar collateral ligament is intact. The cortical outline and joint is well maintained. No evidence of hyper-abduction injury. On the ulnar aspect of the dorsal wrist, the triangular fibrocartilages demonstrates homogenous echogenicity. No evidence of tearing.

Images of the metacarpo-phalangeal joints dorsal and palmar demonstrate no cortical irregularity or destruction. Synovial fluid and/or hypertrophy are/are not noted in the joint margins. Doppler signal to identify synovial hypertrophy was not seen. No A1 pulley hypertrophy or abnormality as seen with trigger finger.

Sample Reports
Knee

Static real-time views in longitudinal and transverse orientation were obtained on this ___ year old male/female. An acoustic stand-off was/was not utilized.

Suprapatellar images demonstrate an intact, fibrillar pattern of the quadriceps tendon. It is not edematous , measuring < 5.0 mm in thickness. The suprapatellar bursa is seen ,but does not exceed 2.5 mm thickness or 22.5 mm length. The patellar tendon is normal (3.0—3.4 mm thickness normal). The prepatellar and infrapatellar subcutaneous bursa are not enlarged due to effusion. The more distal deep infrapatellar bursa is not visualized. No evidence of Osgood –Schlatter's disease. On transverse view, the patellar fat pad is well insonated, and the tibial plateau is smooth with a normal joint margin present.

The lateral collateral ligament is visible at the fibular head attachment, and does not demonstrate sonographic evidence of edema or partial thickness tear. The more superficial biceps femoris tendon is normal.

The medial collateral ligament is normal with a proximal thickness of 3.6-3.8 mm, and a distal thickness of 2.0—2.3 mm. No pes anserine bursal effusion is demonstrated superficial to the MCL tibial attachment . The pes anserine tendon is unremarkable.

Peripheral margins of the medial and lateral menisci are accessible to ultrasound imaging. The medial and lateral menicii demonstrate homogenous echoes of normal fibro-cartilage in the anterior and posterior portions. No evidence of meniscal cysts in peri-articular locations.

Popliteal images are negative for Baker's cyst, vascular abnormality,or mass.

Sample Reports
Ankle and Foot

Static real-time views in longitudinal and transverse orientation were obtained on this ___ year old male/female.

On anterior images, the tibialis anterior, extensor hallucis, and extensor digitorum tendons are hyperechoic,and have normal dense fibrillar pattern. The anterior joint space is approximately 2mm in thickness. No evidence of loose bodies in the joint, or degenerative changes.
At the antero-lateral margin of the ankle, the talo-fibular ligament has no area of non-visualization as seen with tears from inversion injury. The interosseous tibio-fibular ligament is intact,and not inflamed.

Posterior to the lateral malleolus, the calcaneo-fibular ligament is normal. The peroneous longus ,and deeper, peroneous brevis present as normal hyperechoic tendons with dense fibrillar pattern.
The peroneous brevis is attached and intact at the 5th metatarsal base.

The tarsal tunnel structures which include the tibialis posterior, flexor digitorum, flexor hallucis, and the tibial nerve demonstrate normal echogenic tendons, and an ovoid ,hypoechoic nerve.

Achilles tendon long axis image demonstrates a normal fibrillar pattern throughout, from the calcaneal insertion proximally. On short axis it is reniform, and does not have sonographic criteria for inflammation. The retrocalcaneal bursa is not enlarged. No advential bursa present superficial to the tendon. Kager's fat pad is well visualized, and not displaced.
On long axis the plantar fascia is intact and not thicker than 3.5– 4.0 mm. Bursal fluid is noted. Bone spurs on calcaneous are not noted by cortical irregularity or defect.
The distal plantar foot shows normal flexor tendons. The plantar plate ligaments and accessory ligaments present a homogenous interdigital echogenicity, this no hypoechoic mass compatible with neuroma is present.

1359259